H. Anacker · H. D. Weiss · B. Kramann

Endoscopic Retrograde Pancreatico-cholangiography (ERPC)

With 93 Figures

Springer-Verlag
Berlin Heidelberg New York 1977

Professor Dr. HERMANN ANACKER
Dr. HANS-DIETER WEISS
Dr. BERNHARD HEINRICH KRAMANN
Institut für Röntgendiagnostik der Technischen Universität,
Klinikum rechts der Isar,
Ismaninger Str. 22, 8000 München 80

ISBN-13:978-3-642-81090-9 e-ISBN-13:978-3-642-81088-6
DOI: 10.1007/978-3-642-81088-6

Library of Congress Cataloging in Publication Data. Anacker, Hermann, 1917– . Endoscopic retrograde pancreaticocholangiography (ERPC). Bibliography: p. Includes index. 1. Bile-ducts – Radiography. 2. Pancreatic duct – Radiography. 3. Endoscope and endoscopy. I. Weiss, Hans-Dieter, 1938. Joint author. II. Kramann, B., 1940. Joint author. III. Title. [DNLM: 1. Cholangiography. 2. Endoscopy. 3. Pancreas – Radiography. WI800 A532e]. RC847.A5. 616.3′65′0757. 76-50000.

Softcover reprint of the hardcover 1st edition 1977

2123/3130-543210

HOMO
PARS EX TOTO
POSSIBILE STUDENS
ANOMINE SUBMERGENS
MANET GLORIA DEI

Contents

1. **Introduction** 1
   Peroperative Pancreaticography 1
   Terminology 2

2. **The History of Pancreaticography** 3

2.1 Experiments on Pancreaticography by Means of a Balloon Catheter 3
2.2 Experiments on Pancreaticography by Direct Puncture of the Pancreatic Parenchyma 7
2.3 Experiments on Transvenous Pancreaticography 7
2.4 Development of the Endoscopic Retrograde Pancreatico-cholangiography 7

3. **Techniques** 10

3.1 Equipment 10
3.1.1 Endoscopic Equipment 10
3.1.2 Catheters 12
3.1.3 Roentgenologic Equipment 14
3.1.4 Contrast Material 14
3.2 Preparation of the Patient 14
3.3 Technique of ERPC 15
3.3.1 Endoscopy in ERPC 15
3.3.2 Roentgenology in ERPC 20
3.4 Technical Difficulties in ERPC 22

4. **Indications, Contraindications, and Complications** 25

4.1 Indications for ERPC 25
4.2 Contraindications 25
4.3 Hazards, Complications, and Treatment 26

5. **The Normal Retrograde Pancreaticogram** (including anomalies and deformities) 31

5.1 Site of the Papilla of Vater 31
5.2 The Anatomy of the Papilla of Vater 31
5.3 Main Duct and Side Branches of the Pancreas 33
5.4 Width of the Pancreatic Main Duct 38
5.5 Different Types and Variations of the Orifice 40
5.6 The Normal Emptying Process of the Pancreatic Duct . . 44

5.7 Transpapillary Pressure Measurement in the Pancreatic Duct and the Common Bile Duct 46
5.7.1 Method 47
5.7.2 Measuring Errors 48
5.7.3 Characteristic Pressure Tracings 49
5.7.4 Pressure Values in the Pancreatic Duct 51
5.7.5 Pressure Values in the Common Bile Duct 51
5.7.6 Pressure Values in the Duodenum 52

6. The ERPC Roentgenographic Pattern in Changes Due to Age 54

7. The ERPC in Lesions of the Pancreas and the Papilla Duodeni 56

7.1 Annular Pancreas 56
7.2 Chronic Pancreatitis, Chronic Relapsing Pancreatitis, Calculous Pancreatitis 57
7.3 Necrotizing Lesions and Pseudocysts 67
7.4 Papillary Stenosis and Papillary Spasm 74
7.5 Benign Tumors of the Pancreas 78
7.6 Carcinoma of the Pancreas 79
7.7 Papillary Carcinoma 91
7.8 Metastases of Tumors to the Pancreas 94
7.9 Posttraumatic Conditions of the Pancreas 95
7.10 Postoperative Conditions of the Pancreas 95

8. ERPC in Diseases of the Biliary Tract 97

8.1 Primary Sclerosing Cholangitis 97
8.2 Secondary Sclerosing Cholangitis and Postoperative Conditions of the Biliary Tract 97
8.3 Calculous Disease of the Bile Ducts and the Gallbladder 100
8.4 Carcinoma of the Bile Ducts and Carcinoma of the Liver 101
8.5 Stenosis of the Common Bile Duct Secondary to Diseases of Pancreas and Liver 102

9. Correlation of ERPC with Other Roentgenologic Examinations of the Pancreas 105

10. Conclusion 110

11. References 111

12. Subject Index 121

1. Introduction

The roentgenologic visualization of excretory ducts of a secreting organ is a longe-stablished diagnostic method in roentgenology. For a long time, radiologists have felt the need to establish a method for filling the excretory duct system of the pancreas with contrast material, in the way that intravenous retrograde urography is used to diagnose pathologic changes such as displacement of the renal collecting system or of the urethra. This need to establish a method became more urgent the more the pancreas resisted conventional roentgenologic clinical diagnostic methods. From time to time in peroperative or postoperative cholangiography mostly incomplete reflux into the pancreatic duct in 10–14% was observed (Stiller, 1948; San Julian und Pascual y Megias, 1952; Wapshaw, 1955; Bergkvist und Seldinger, 1957). However, there was no possibility of obtaining reliable and complete opacification of the pancreatic duct.

Peroperative Pancreaticography

It was in 1951 when Léger and Arway achieved this goal, though only by surgery. It should be mentioned that, when performing their first peroperative examination, these French surgeons already had the impression, that cannulation of the pancreatic duct was easier than cannulation of the common bile duct. This observation has been confirmed by hundreds of examinations after ERPC had been established for several years; however, up till now this phenomenon has not been sufficiently explained.

During the following years, peroperative pancreaticography developed into a routine examination, above all by Doubilet et al. (1955), Mercadier and Hepp (1956), Fritsch (1957), Vosschulte (1961, 1962, 1963), Vosschulte and Wagner (1968), and Léger (1964). There were three different variations: (1) puncture of the pancreatic main duct through the parenchyma, (2) descending pancreaticography after partial pancreatectomy of the tail, (3) transduodenal cannulation of the papilla of Vater after the duodenum has been incised. This examination could only be performed peroperatively, limited to those cases where surgery was indicated, i.e., mainly to chronic pancreatitis with stenoses and to pancreatic carcinoma. Reports were published on exact observations concerning the changes of the duct system, secondary to chronic pancreatitis, and to carcinoma; and many of those observations are still valid today. These findings were completed by means of detailed studies on the excretory duct system, filled with contrast medium in a resected specimen (Clairmont, 1920; Kleitsch, 1955; Smanio, 1955; Szebök and Mészaros, 1957; Gualdi and Messe, 1959, 1960; Fritsch, 1957; Birnstingel, 1959; Millbourn, 1959, 1960; Anacker, 1961, 1967; Warter and Weill et al., 1965; Hentschel, 1968).

All these studies show that roentgenologic visualization of the pancreatic duct system is a good diagnostic key for assessing the changes of the inner structure of the gland in chronic pancreatitis and of deformations in pancreatic carcinoma. The most important aim, however, roentgenologic demonstration of the pancreatic ducts without surgery, had not yet been reached. When the value of this examination had been proved, attempts were made to establish a method of filling the duct system with contrast medium, a method that presents less hazards and discomfort to the patient.

Terminology

The word "pancreatography" usually defines the parenchymal phase, i.e., the visualization of the parenchyma during arteriography. The same term had been used, also, for radiologic demonstration of the entire organ in pneumostratigraphy. On the other hand, the surgical terminology defines "pancreaticojejunostomy" as a surgical anastomosis between the pancreatic duct and the jejunum. Therefore, the authors agree with Burwood et al., that the term "pancreaticography" seems to be the most suitable one for the visualization of the pancreatic duct.

2. The History of Pancreaticography

2.1 Experiments on Pancreaticography by Means of a Balloon Catheter

The first experimental studies concerning retrograde filling of the pancreatic duct were made in 1949–1955. They were based on the theory that an acute hemorrhagic pancreatitis might be caused by a reflux of duodenal juice into the pancreatic duct, as had been observed by Pfeffer et al. (1957) in animal experiments. The authors had studied this problem on resected specimens consisting of the descending (1953) part of the duodenum and the gland. According to Bartelheimer (1953) they introduced a duodenal tube with three channels and two balloons into the duodenum. The balloons were inflated until sufficient tightening was obtained. Then a highly diluted barium suspension was infused into the channel that ended between the two balloons. The authors never saw a reflux from the duodenum to the pancreas, even when the pressure was elevated to the maximum. In 1955, Gaylis and Gunn, when using this technique, though using diodone for transduodenal cholangiography in five postmortem studies, obtained the same negative results.

The negative results were supposed to be due to the oblique course of the prepapillary segment of the common bile duct in the duodenal wall with consecutive tightening by the duodenal folds, which especially in high pressures, may obstruct the papilla. However, in two patients with papillary insufficiency and consecutive pneumatosis of the bile ducts, Gaylis and Gunn were able to provoke a reflux into the common bile duct under the same experimental conditions. These authors supposed that the regular absence of a duodeno-biliary reflux in the living patient might be due to an increased tonus of the sphincter of Oddi, as well as the above-mentioned mechanism that had been shown in the postmortem studies. In 1955, Greenfield et. al. tried to overcome the neurogenic factor by means of pharmacodynamic agents. They did not succeed, however, in obtaining reliable and reproducible successful results. In 1966, Schmarsow, using amylnitrite, ether, or trinitine, confirmed the negative outcome of such studies, as well as the author's results, who had studied the effect of diluted hydrochloric acid in order to decrease the tonus of the sphincter of the Oddi. Later, Waldron et. al. (1967), Doppmann et. al. (1967), as well as Waldron et al. (1968), and Rosenbaum et al. (1971) carried out animal experiments with the doubleballoon tube, which was introduced orally or by surgery. By simultaneous relaxation of the duodenum and the sphincter of Oddi, or by transvenous injections of secretin and cholecystokininpancreozymin, they succeeded in provoking a reflux in a higher percentage. The reflux into the pancreatic duct could be observed more often than a reflux into the bile duct. However, since this technique, combined with the application of secretin and cholecystokinin provoked acute pancreatitis, this method could not be applied to man.

On the other hand, when using relaxers with less imminent danger of pancreatitis, the filling of the pancreatic duct system was highly inconstant with regard to incidence, time, and duodenal pressure. No means was found to provoke a reliable reflux in low duodenal pressure. In 1972 Waldron tried to apply this technique to man, a technique that had been successful in a certain percentage of animal experiements. These experiments had a dissapointing outcome. In 18 patients a retrograde filling of the pancreatic ducts could never be observed. Only three patients showed a temporary partial filling of the neighboring segment of the main duct. All three patients had a duodenal diverticulum. Furthermore, in one of these patients there was an elevation of serum amylase as a sign of a pancreatic lesion.

The second way to obtain a preoperative visualization of the pancreatic duct system can be realized by provoking a biliary-pancreatic reflux. This idea arose in 1953 when roentgenologic demonstrations of the bile duct became feasible by means of transvenous application of contrast material. Thus, in 1955 the authors tried to obtain a biliary pancreatic reflux in autopsy specimen. An inflatable balloon was introduced into the duodenum and was placed just in front of the papilla of Vater. Then with alternating pressure, a water-soluble or oily contrast agent (Urographin 40%, Joduron, Jodipin) was injected into the ligated common bile duct. Thirty-four studies on eight autopsy specimens showed the results shown in Table 1.

Table 1

Balloon pressure	Injection pressure		
	High	Medium	Slight
High	− + + +	+ − +	+ − + − −
Medium	+		−
Slight	− +	−	− +
Without balloon	+ − − − −	− − − − −	− − − − −

This demonstrated that, except on a single case, the biliary-pancreatic reflux could never be provoked unless an inflated balloon was placed in front of the papilla. In this exceptional case, the resected specimen presented a 1.5 mm-long common duct, that might have been the cause for the reflux. But even in this case, a reflux could only be provoked

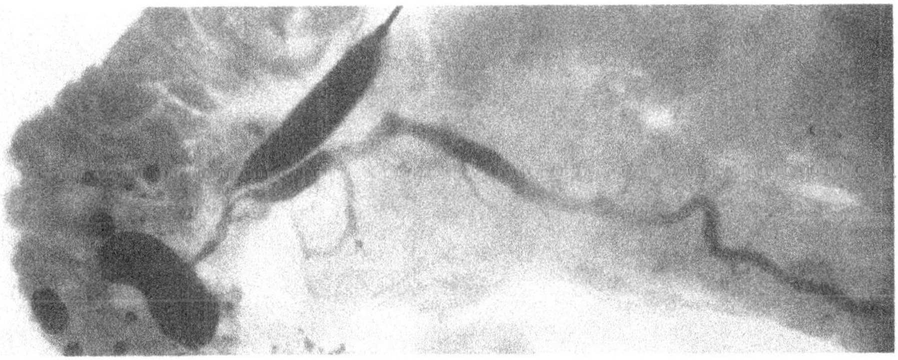

Fig. 1. Biliary-pancreatic reflux in resected specimen. 1.5 mm long common prepapillary duct segment of common bile duct and of Wirsung's duct. Extremely high injection pressure. Slight injection pressure could not provoke a reflux

by extreme injection pressure (Fig. 1). This finding corresponds well with retrograde filling of the pancreatic duct as it can be observed in peroperative or postoperative cholangiography.

However, when the papilla is tightened by a balloon, a biliary-pancreatic reflux occurs more often, and the higher the injection pressure, the more the balloon is inflated (Fig. 2). Yet, this biliary-pancreatic reflux was far from being reproduced regularly.

In one anatomical specimen with a duodenal diverticulum, in which the common bile duct had been filled, the authors observed filling of the pancreatic main duct via the bile duct after the orifice in the

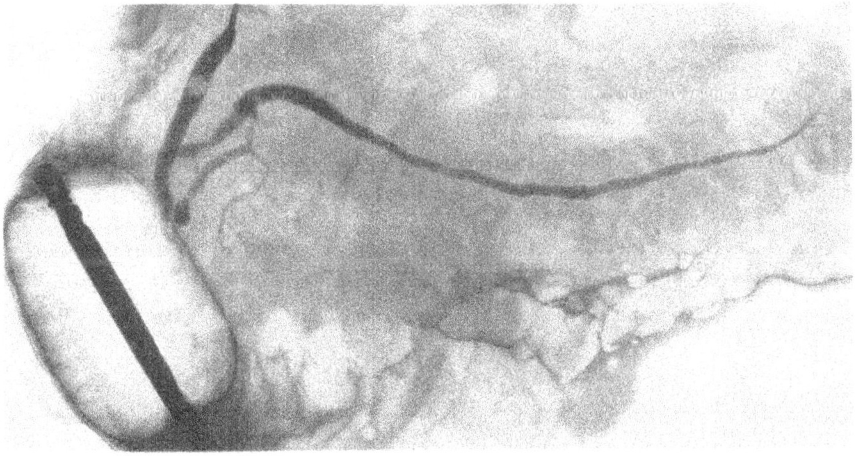

Fig. 2. Biliary-pancreatic reflux after papilla has been tightened by inflated balloon in resected specimen. Reflux could not be reproduced without balloon, even when injection pressure was high

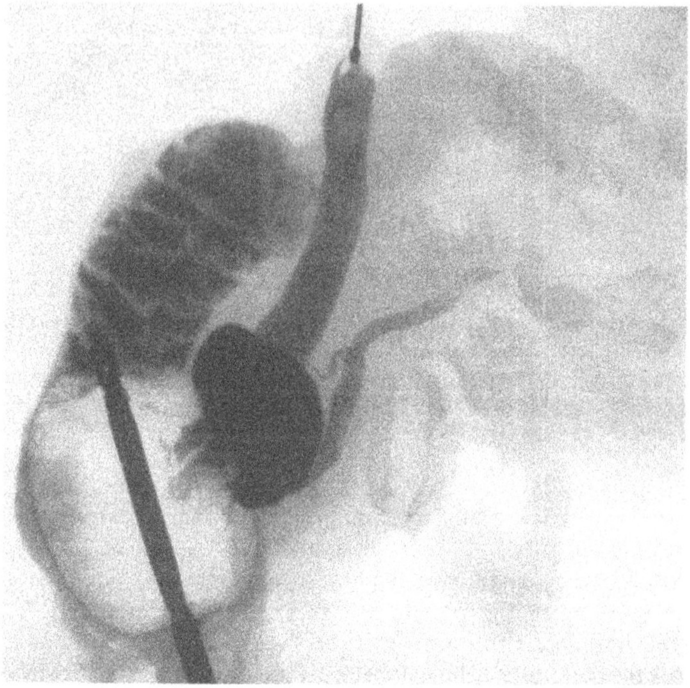

Fig. 3. Biliary-pancreatic reflux after injection of contrast material into common bile duct with simultaneous tightening of papilla by inflated balloon. Resected specimen, showing common opening of bile duct and pancreatic duct into duodenal diverticulum. During injection of dye reflux could be demonstrated only after diverticulum had been filled first. Without tightening of balloon no reflux could be provoked, even in higher injection pressure

duodenum had been tightened by an inflated balloon. Thus, a biliary-pancreatic reflux was provoked (Fig. 3). In view of the often discussed role of the duodenal diverticulum in the development of chronic pancreatitis, it may be of clinical interest that, in a diverticulum, the pancreatic duct can be filled by reflux from the bile duct, if the pressure in the bile duct is elevated.

Hence, clinically relevant use of retrograde filling of the pancreatic duct system by means of a biliary-pancreatic reflux after transvenous cholangiography is not to be expected, since the filling pressure in the common bile duct cannot be sufficiently obtained, quite apart from the risk that is inherent in a biliary-pancreatic reflux.

This conclusion was supported by studies on patients. A reflux of contrast material from the common bile duct into the pancreatic duct after intravenous application of Biligrafin could never be provoked by an inflated balloon positioned in front of the papilla and simultaneous application of hypophysine, leading to contraction of the gallbladder, which increases the bile duct pressure.

2.2 Experiments on Pancreaticography by Direct Puncture of the Pancreatic Parenchyma

When water-soluble contrast material is injected directly into the parenchyma of a resected specimen, one can observe filling of the smallest branches in the vicinity of a diffuse opacification of the parenchyma (Fig. 4a). The authors succeeded only once (in 1963) in filling the main duct by means of such a blind puncture (Fig. 4b).

Experiments of this kind have been, and may still be, of quite theoretical interest, for it may be rather dubious if one will ever try to puncture the pancreas in vivo. Nevertheless, from the historical point of view, with regard to the various attempts to get a preoperative demonstration of the pancreatic duct system, it may be of some interest to know, that in a certain percentage there is a theoretical possibility of directly puncturing the pancreatic gland.

2.3 Experiments on Transvenous Pancreaticography

In 1963, Silverman and Hill tried to fill the pancreatic duct system with contrast medium by transvenous cholecystography. After having administered 40 ml Cholografin intravenously for opacification of the gallbladder, they injected 15–20 mg of morphine sulfate combined with 1 mg of Lorfan tartrate intravenously followed by an intravenous application of 75 μ cholecystokinin 25 min later. During the following 45 min they made abdominal plain films, combined with tomography. These authors could not visualize the pancreatic duct system in any of their patients.

In experiments on animals, Ledoux-Lebard et al. (1964) observed an opacification of the pancreas after intravenous injection of Erythrosine B. This opacification could be demonstrated on substraction images. The duct itself, however, could not be visualized in any case. These authors believe that pancreatic opacification with Erythrosine B in man will only be feasible if the very complicated experimental conditions necessary in animal experiments, can be simplified. In fact, there are no reports of application of this transvenous method in man.

2.4 Development of the Endoscopic Retrograde Pancreaticocholangiography

In 1965, Rabinov and Simon followed a completely new course by trying to cannulate the papilla of Vater directly from the duodenum. For this purpose they used a special elastic tube. At the end of the tube there was a basket-like construction of rods that could be spread. A guidable cannula was passed through this basket. The tube was

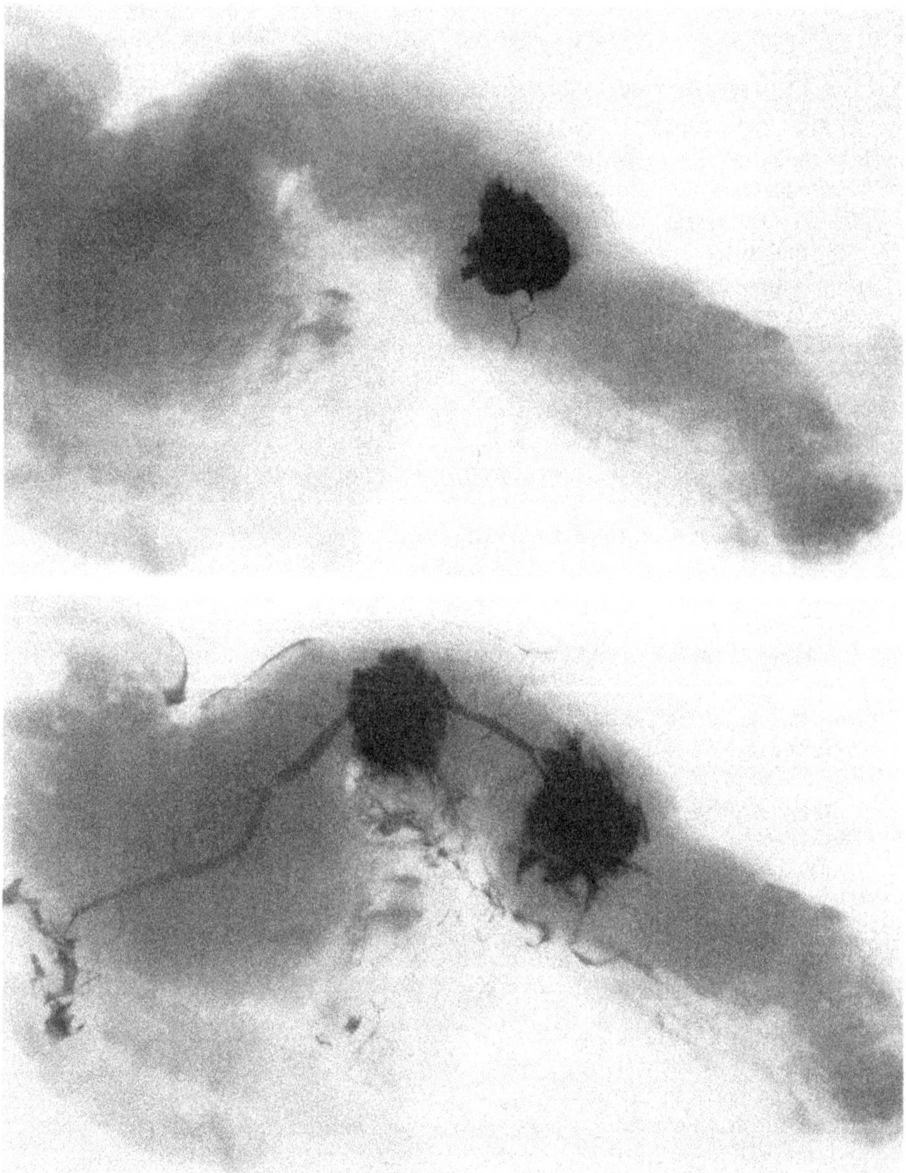

a

b

Fig. 4a and b. Direct puncture of a resected specimen with direct injection of contrast material. Escape of dye from depot into small side branch (a). A second puncture of another region succeeded in direct filling of Wirsung's duct (b)

introduced perorally. At the level of the papilla the basket was spread and one tried to enter the opening with the cannula. The cannulation was controlled only by fluoroscopic monitoring. Consequently, the yield was rather poor. Of eight cases, cannulation succeeded only once. However, the decisive and new factor in these experiments is that for the following periods a promising road had been shown by instrumental cannulation of the papilla.

Following this road, McCune et al. (1968) introduced the EDER-fiberduodenoscope, which allowed a direct view of the papilla of Vater. Instead of the uncertain fluoroscopic control, one could demonstrate and cannulate the papilla under direct vision, and the cannulation rate of the pancreatic duct system could be elevated up to 25%. McCune et al. substituted the spreadable basket by an inflatable balloon in order to keep the tip of the instrument away from the duodenal wall. All patients tolerated the examinations without any hazards.

With the introduction of the fiberendoscope for cannulation of the papilla under direct endoscopic control, the last step was made toward reproducible pancreaticography, a method that made surgical intervention for cannulation unnecessary. Rapid progress in techniques of fiberendoscopy for duodenoscopy put this method on a sound basis. This is true, above all, for Japan where Oi et al. (1969), Oi et al. (1970), Takagi et al. (1970), Ogohsi et al. (1970), and Kozu (1970) reported on the first successful pancreaticographies and cholangiographies with the improved Machida and Olympus instruments. These instruments did not need a basket or a balloon for keeping the tip of the instrument away from the duodenal wall. Their special advantages were the improved optical systems, the flexibility of the tip, which allowed better maneuvering and better handling, as well as the large instrument channels that allowed forceps biopsy or brush biopsy. While Takagi et al. preferred general anesthesia, Oi et al. performed the examination in local anesthesia of the larynx. By using this fiberduodenoscope, the rate of successful cannulation and roentgenologic visualization of the pancreatic main duct and the bile ducts was increased up to 70%.

In Germany this method was introduced by Demling and Classen (1970) and Anacker et al. (1971), in France by Jeanpierre et al. (1971), in England by Cotten et al. (1972), in Hungary by Safrany (1972), and in Switzerland by Deyhle et al. (1972). It was Classen above all who developed the technique that may be regarded as the standard method of ERPC.

3. Techniques

In order to yield the most diagnostic information, perfect practice of all parts of the technique is mandatory, as well as maximal demonstration of the pancreatic and the biliary duct systems. This percentage increases with the authors' experience as Table 2 shows.

Table 2. Experience in ERCP and successful cannulation rate

Number of cases	Cannulation rate
1 – 100	56%
100 – 200	74%
200 – 500	93%
500 – 1,000	94%

3.1 Equipment

3.1.1 Endoscopic Equipment

In 1969 and 1970 the only available fiberduodenoscope, the Machida F.D.S. duodenoscope, was introduced. It seemed well-suited for ERPC. As Takagi and Oi had already shown, the instrument allowed endoscopy of the papilla, cannulation, and injection of contrast medium. Yet, the instrument had some shortcomings that obviously complicated the examination. The infinitely variable focus revealed, at least in the authors' experience, to be a drawback, for respiratory movements, movements due to pulsations of arteries and occasional peristalsis, forced the examiner to incessantly adjust the focus.

The enormous flexibility of the endoscopic tube, which, compared to the former rigid instruments appeared to be epoch-making, turned out to be another shortcoming, since the obvious loss of the straight-on shearing strength may seriously impede the passage of the pyloric channel in lateral-viewing endoscopes. Yet, some investigators, especially in Japan, still prefer this instrument on account of its excellent optical system, as well as its larger instrument channel.

Since 1971, the authors have used the Olympus duodenoscope, which has proved to be excellent for ERPC (Fig. 5). Like the Machida duodenoscopes, the Olympus fiberduodenoscope JFB I and JFB II are equipped with a side-viewing optical system. The instrument is 1,520 mm long with an effective working length of 1,370 mm. The

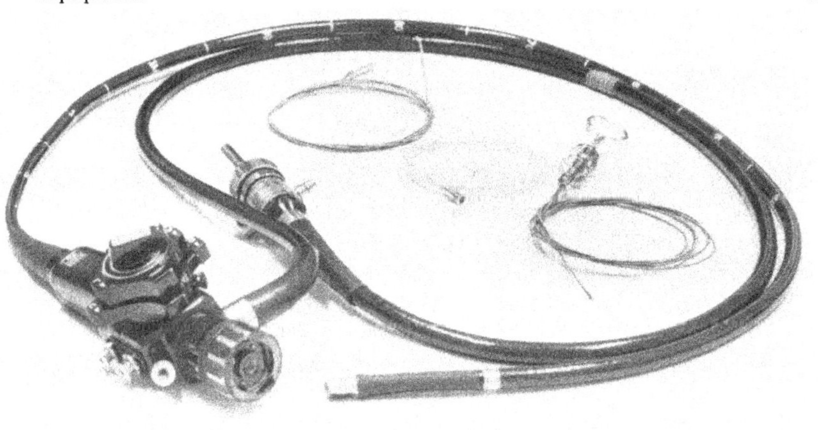

Fig. 5. Olympus duodenoscope JFB with polyethylene cannula, biopsy forceps, and cytology brush

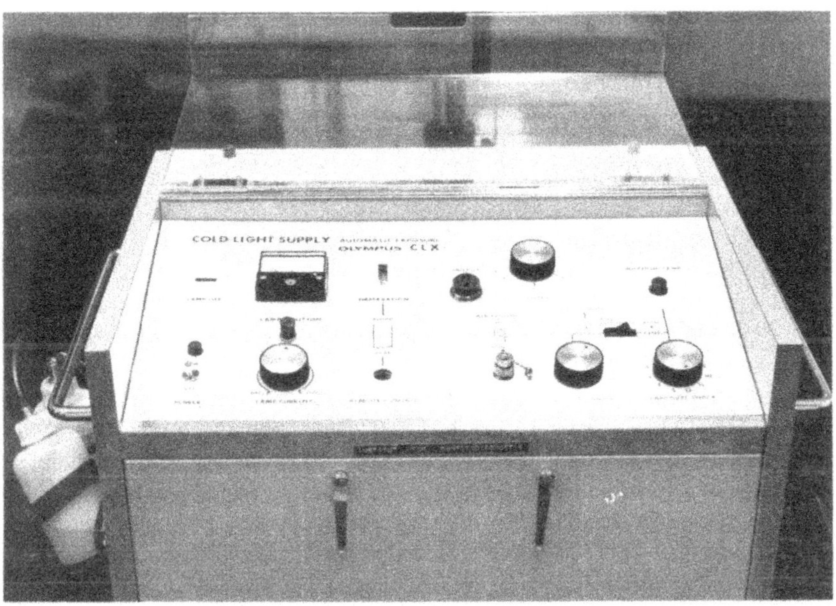

Fig. 6. The "big" Olympus cold light supply model CLX is highly suited for endoscopy, cinematography, and photography

outer diameter of the insertion tube is 10 mm. The 46-mm-long bending section has a four-way angulation mechanism (120° up, 120° down, 90° right, and 90° left). The forceps-raiser enables the operator to adjust the elevation angle of the cannula, cytology brush, or biopsy forceps. The maximum elevation angle is 80°.

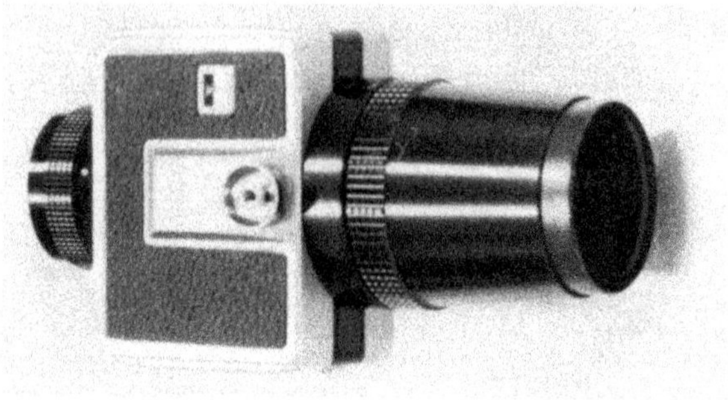

Fig. 7. Olympus mini-camera SC 16/2, very handy and performs automatic exposure photography

The optical system proved to be highly suited for ERPC. The fixed focus with a range of observation from 5–60 mm guarantees constant optical conditions in spite of the indirect or direct movements of the descending duodenum. The 65° angle of the field of view is sufficient. These advantages, as well as the flexibility of the angulation mechanism, are completed by the excellent traceability. Thus, the slightest movements, such as rotation of the control unit, are sufficiently transmitted to the tip of the instrument, while the eyepiece of the instrument is leaned closely against the operators face for finest movement control. In this way fine adjusting movements, which are essential for cannulation, can be performed.

For illumination, several cold light source models such as the CLE, CLS, and the CLX are available. They guarantee sufficient illumination for all endoscopic phases (Fig. 6). The authors prefer the high intensity cold light model CLX, which seems to be specially suited for cinematography or photography documentation. The automatic camera SC 16/2 is an appropriate optical accessory. It combines the advantages of being small, handy, and light (Fig. 7). This camera performs excellent automatic exposure photography. Furthermore, in contrast to the PEN/F camera, this device has the advantage of presenting a slightly magnified endoscopic view, so that a trained operator can perform the whole endoscopic examination with the attached camera ready to shoot.

3.1.2 Catheters

In principle, cannulation of the papilla can be performed with any catheter that can pass the instrument channel and whose tip can be preshaped. Yet, certain materials such as teflon or polyethylene seem to have certain advantages. Olympus polyaethylene catheters with distance markers at the tip are available. These catheters are useful and allow the endoscopist to get sufficient cannulation rates. However, since the tip is rather flexible and unstable it may sometimes complicate cannulation. For routine cannulation the authors use a metal-tipped polyethylene catheter, which has been made according to their proposal. The metal tip, which can serve as a good landmark in the roentgenograms, is screwed on to the catheter. The catheter has an outer diameter of 1.5 mm, and it should be at least 2,500 mm long in order to allow the examiner to get the syringe sufficiently away from the instrument. The catheter is large enough to allow suction with or without combined stimulation of the pancreas, as well as reliable pressure control of the biliary or pancreatic duct system. For deep cannulation of the duct systems, one can pass guide wires through the catheter.

If opacification of one of the diagnostic relevant duct systems fails, the authors use a Vygon balloon catheter. This angiography catheter has an inflatable balloon close to the tip that allows the examiner to anchor the catheter tip in the papilla. In preliminary experiments with this cannulation technique on resected duodenal and pancreatic specimens, the authors found an increased frequency of successful filling of the biliary duct system when the catheter was anchored in the ampulla of Vater by means of the inflated balloon. The authors tried to stretch the terminal segments of the two ducts by slightly pulling back the catheter in order to obtain more propitious angulation deflections of the intrapapillary terminal duct segments.

Another means for demonstrating the bile ducts has been found by cannulation of the papilla with a tube that can be passed through the catheter. The tip of the inner catheter is preshaped with a curve directed cranially. After cannulation of the papilla with the outer catheter, the inner preshaped catheter is advanced and then retracted, so that the preshaped tip glides into the opening of the common bile duct, which is situated cranially.

For routine diagnosis the authors' principally use the two catheters mentioned first, since the pancreatic duct system can be sufficiently visualized in 86–90% of cases. In the authors, case material the bile ducts could be visualized in 74%, regarding the fact that dilatation of the bile ducts secondary to biliary lesions leads to an increased filling rate.

For *biopsy,* Olympus devices such as biopsy forceps and brushes are available as well as a Meditech nylon brush. This latter brush presents some advantages. Although the biopsy forceps provides sufficient results, it seems to grasp too superficially. Thus neoplasms overlayed by an inflammatory process may escape histologic examination. The shortcoming of the Olympus brush is its large caliber, which does not allow the operator to pass the brush through the instrument channel together with a protective catheter. In order to prevent the cytologic material from being stripped off, the brush is only retracted through the instrument channel together with the fiberendocope. Thus, a second brush biopsy would necessitate another endoscopic examination.

This shortcoming can be avoided by using the Meditech brush, which has been developed especially for brush biopsy of other organs, such as the bronchi or the renal collecting system. This brush can be pushed through the normal ERPC catheter and it can be retracted together with the catheter. Thus, repeated brush biopsy can be performed while the endoscope is left in place. Simultaneous opacification of the pancreatic duct and brush biopsy of the suspected area are feasible. To prevent injuries to the duct wall in the proximal segments one can push the catheter forward into the suspected segment by means of Teflon-coated guide wire. After removal of the guide wire and introduction of the brush, selective brush biopsy can be performed.

3.1.3 Roentgenologic Equipment

Theoretically, ERPC can be performed with basic equipment including an X-ray table with a tube and a fluoroscopic screen in one plane only.

However, prevention of possible hazards secondary to overfilling of the pancreatic duct system with acinar and even periacinar opacification, necessitates television fluoroscopic control with high resolving power. The operator able to assess the filling degree can pinpoint the quantity of dye necessary for sufficient diagnostic information. The diagnostic yield constitutes another factor that argues in favor of high quality fluoroscopic monitoring since the controlled opacification of the main duct and the side branches of first and second degree increases considerably the diagnostic yield. On the other hand, a false negative diagnosis due to insufficient opacification of the duct system can be avoided much better.

3.1.4 Contrast Material

The authors use Conray 60 (iodthalamic acid), which does not contain sodium saline. It has the advantage of being less viscous than other contrast materials. Furthermore, as Manegold (1974) demonstrated, there is a statistically relevant less higher elevation of serum lipase secondary to ERPC performed with Conray 60. Less radiopaque contrast agents increase the hazards of overfilling. The quantity of the injected contrast agent plays a less important role since the catheter does not completely tighten the papilla so that a certain amount of "surplus" dye flows back into the duodenum.

3.2 Preparation of the Patient

As in every endoscopic examination of the upper digestive tract, the patient's stomach must be empty for ERPC as well. In the individual case the examination can be performed 3 hours after the patient has had his last meal, provided that there is no disease that may hinder the normal emptying of the stomach and of the duodenum. If ERPC is performed in the afternoon, the authors let the patient have his breakfest in the morning. Thus, secretion of gastric juice of the empty stomach may be reduced. The patient, 15 min prior to examination, is given an intramuscular injection of 10 mg Psyquil (triflupromacine) combined with 0.5 mg atropine. Triflupromacine reduces peristalses while yielding sufficient tonus of the gastric and duodenal wall. Vasovagal reflexes, which may be induced by endoscopy and insufflation of air, are suppressed with atropine, which furthermore reduces secretion of gastric juice. Immediately prior to examination, 50 mg of Dolantin (meperidine) are given transvenously.

Frothing in the duodenum can be suppressed by an antifoamer—silicone preparations such as Endoparactol (dimethylpolysiloxan)—that can be administered orally before introducing the instrument or passed down the instrument channel. For local anesthesia of the larynx, Novesine spray is given by the authors immediately prior to examination.

3.3 Technique of ERPC

3.3.1 Endoscopy in ERPC

Introduction of the Instrument

For endoscopic examination of the stomach and the descending duodenum, the patient should be positioned on his left side or in the prone position. Thus, the gastric juice accumulates in the fornix ventriculi or along the major curvature, while the air collects along the lesser curvature, the antrum, the duodenal bulb, and the descending part of the duodenum.

The duodenoscope is introduced with its tip directed upward to the ceiling. The patient should be encouraged to swallow the instrument actively, thus one can reduce considerably the risk of perforating the recessus piriformis, a well-known endoscopic complication. In any case, the examiner should avoid introducing the instrument by force. An elastic resistance must not be roughly overcome.

The potential risk of esophageal diverticuli or stenoses should lead the examiner to avoid force when passing the instrument through the esophagus and the cardia. In any case, it is better to stop the examination when the esophageal passage present difficulties and to repeat endoscopy, after having otherwise cleared up the esophageal condition, than to expose the patient to an unnecessary danger of perforation. The endoscopic examination begins after the instrument has reached the stomach. The view is directed towards the lesser curvature, which can be easily differentiated from the other parts of the stomach, especially from the greater curvature, due to the fact that the lesser curvature presents an almost parallel course of its mucosal folds.

The examiner may encounter difficulties in cases of cascade-shaped stomachs. In these conditions the instrument may occasionally be trapped in the dorsally overhanging fundus and by further pushing

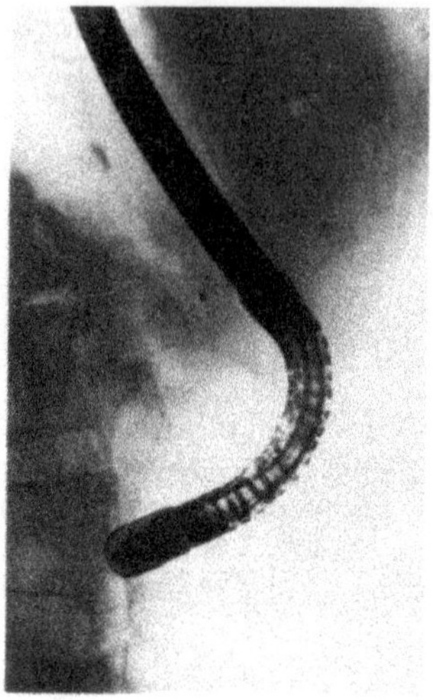
b
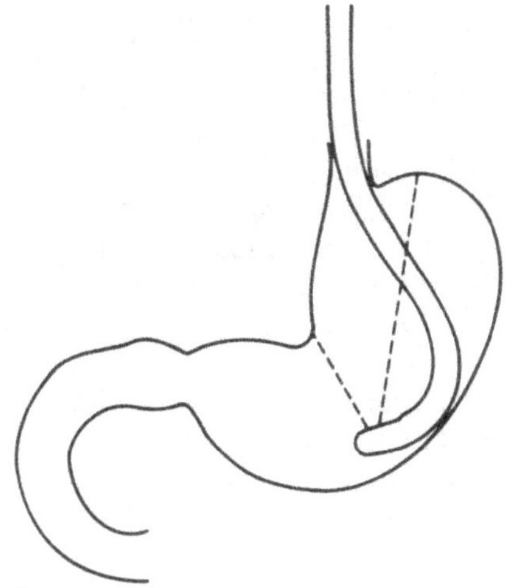
c

Fig. 8a–c. (a see p. 21). Endoscopic view of lesser curvature. Though the stomach is dilated by insufflated air, fold of angulus is still distinct. Behind it view is directed backward to the instrument. (b) Roentgenologic aspect of position of instrument, when endoscopic view is directed toward fold of angulus, the lesser curvature and back to instrument toward cardia. (c) Schematic demonstration of position of instrument and of field of view in stomach, according to endoscopic and roentgenologic aspect

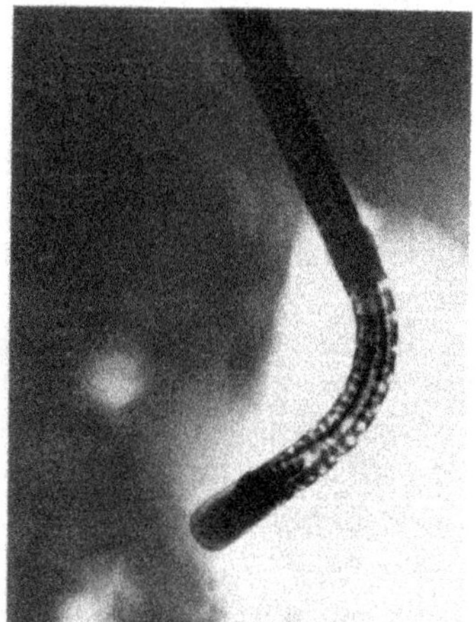
b
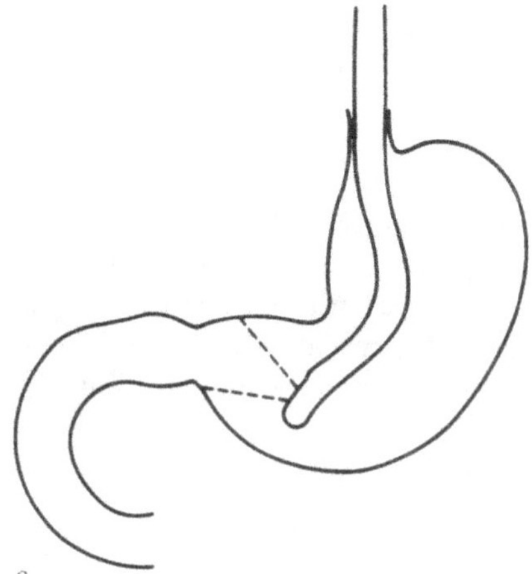
c

Fig. 9a–c. (a see p. 21). Optic approaches pylorus with tip still bent caudally. In this position it is not possible to pass pyloric channel. (b) The instrument is pushed forward with tip bent caudally. View is directed toward prepyloric part of antrum and pyloric channel. Optic, which can be seen on radiogram, is directed toward pyloric channel. (c) Schematic demonstration of most frequent position of instrument, when view is directed toward pyloric channel of the endoscope the distal segment may loop upward. Apart from the less imminent danger of perforation of the gastric wall there is a greater risk that the tip of the instrument may slip into the cardia.

As a rule, dilatation of the cardia causes a sudden severe pain. Of 1,500 endoscopic examinations the authors observed this complication in two patients. In both cases the tip of the duodenoscope was easily drawn back under television fluoroscopic control. Wiendl reports on a similar case, in which it was not possible to draw back the instrument since its tip had been introduced in the cardia in a sharp angle. The endoscope could only be stretched and pulled back into the stomach by laparatomy.

Under normal conditions the instrument is pushed along the major curvature down to the antrum with its optic directed toward the lesser curvature. Constant position control is of utmost importance. The insufflation of air should be kept to a minimum because overdilatation of the stomach causes hyperperistalsis of the stomach and of the duodenum, which may hinder the pyloric passage and cannulation of the papilla. When the instrument has reached the angle of the lesser curvature, the endoscopic view is directed forward toward the antrum as well as backward to the corpus and fornix ventriculi (Fig. 8a–c).

Now the endoscopist tries to get a face-on view of the pyloric channel, which can be achieved with the side-viewing optical system by bending the tip of the instrument caudally. In this position the instrument is advanced toward the pyloric channel as close as possible (Fig. 9a–c). When the instrument is positioned immediately before the pyloric channel, the tip is stretched and blindly pushed forward into the duodenal bulb. When the tip of the bulb is reached, one can generally feel a certain resistance to the fiberscope (Fig. 10a, b).

Although endoscopic examination of the duodenal bulb can be performed with a sideward viewing instrument, it is generally difficult and time-consuming to keep the optic sufficiently away from the mucosa. To avoid unnecessary inflation of air into the duodenum, bulboscopy should be done after pancreaticocholangiography has been performed.

In this position the whole instrument is turned clockwise 180°, while the tip of the instrument is bent caudally with its optic directed toward the descending part of the duodenum.

In some medical centers it is customary to introduce the instrument with the optic directed downward to the floor. When passing through the stomach the tip glides along the lesser curvature, while the optic is directed toward the major curvature.

In this technique it is not necessary to turn the instrument when passing through the duodenal bulb, since the optic is already directed caudally when passing the pyloric channel and the duodenal bulb. Sometimes it may be impossible to push the instrument forward along the major curvature toward the pyloric channel. In these cases the instrument may loop in the body of the stomach close to the lesser

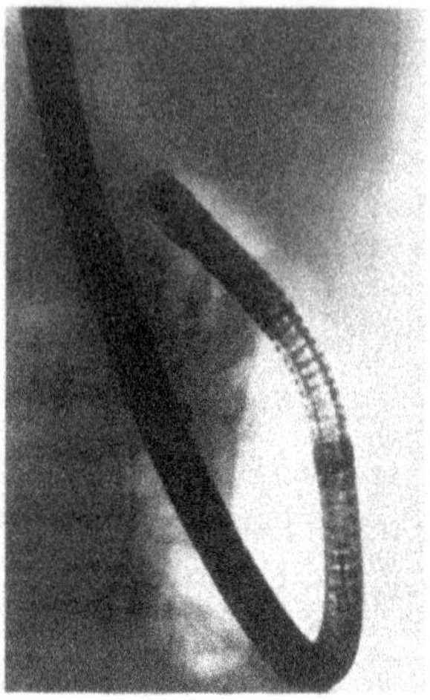
a

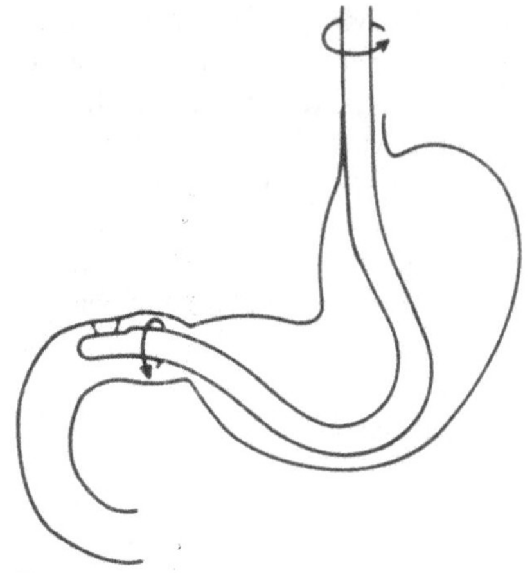
b

Fig. 10. (a) After having passed pyloric channel, instrument tip is in duodenal bulb. Optic is close to duodenal wall. In this position it is often impossible to get a good endoscopic view. (b) Drawing demonstrates position of instrument tip and optic in duodenal bulb

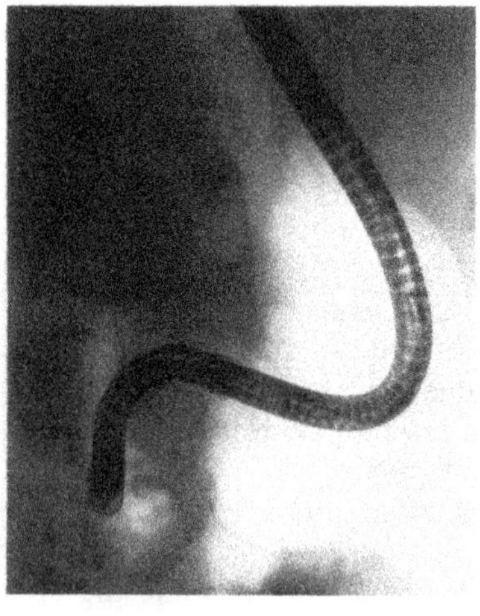
b

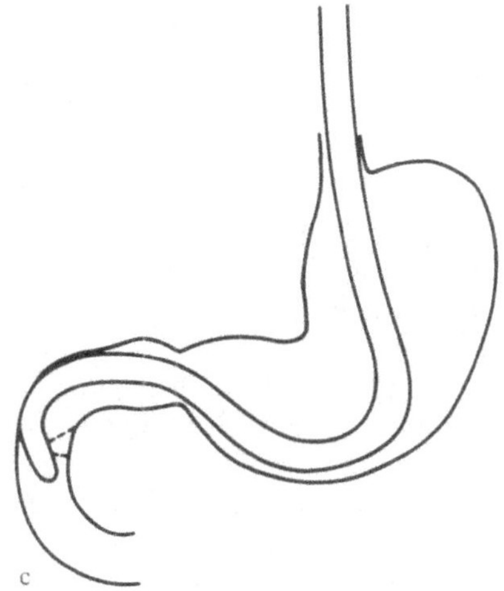
c

Fig. 11a–c. (a see p. 21). After having turned instrument 180° and after slight downward bending of tip, examiner gets endoscopic view into descending part of duodenum. Kerckring's folds can be recognized. (b) Roentgenologic demonstration of instrument's position. Instrument has been turned clockwise 180°. Tip is already bent downward. (c) The field of view is already partially directed toward papillary region

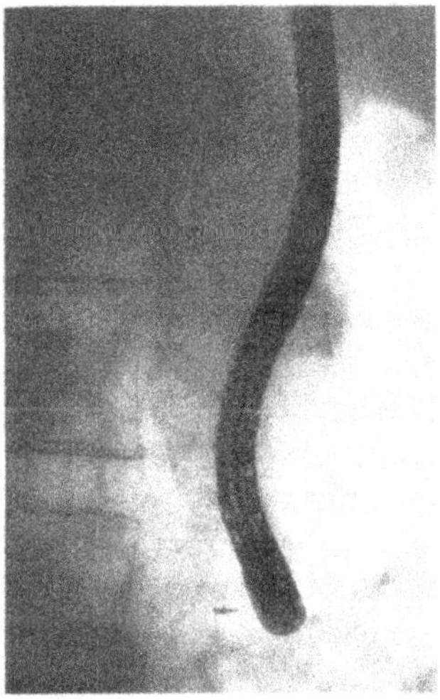

Fig. 12. Radiologic demonstration of straightened instrument. This position guarantees best maneuverability, especially for rotating movements; one can look back to instrument in fornix and corpus ventriculi

curvature with its tip gliding along the major curvature. Thus, when passing the pyloric channel in a fairly exact inverted position, the optic is directed caudally and the endoscopist can look into the descending part of the duodenum without having turned the instrument. Nevertheless, for better control of the instrument it may be advisable to turn it clockwise under fluoroscopic control.

When the instrument has been turned and bent caudally in the duodenal bulb, the tip of the instrument is often immediately in front of the papilla (Fig. 11a–c). Yet, in this position the instrument may strain the lower part of the stomach and the duodenal bulb and stimulate increased peristalsis. Furthermore, the mobility of the instrument is markedly restricted due to the double bending of the insertion tube; rotation is above all restrained and the examiner may encounter difficulties in providing the close face-on papillary view required for cannulation. For these reasons it may be advisable to stretch the instrument by drawing it back. As a rule, when retracting the instrument, the tip pushes forward deeper into the descending part of the duodenum (Fig. 12). In this position fluoroscopic monitoring may be helpful in orientation, for one cannot decide endoscopically, how far the tip of the duodenoscope is positioned in the descending duodenum. All segments of the second and third duodenum present a similar endoscopic aspect. One can distinguish the circular Kerckring's folds presenting a reddish and homogeneous surface. Suspicious changes should be cleared up. Depositions upon the mucosa should be washed away or cleared by forceps or brush biopsy.

Now that the tip of the instrument is situated caudally from the papilla, the whole instrument must be slowly retracted. It is important to obtain a good view of the medial wall of the descending duodenum by continously adjusting the field of view. If the endoscopist is standing exactly in front of the universal cord, the medial wall of the duodenum appears at the lower margin of the field of view.

It is important to bring the instrument in this position, unless the papilla may not appear in the small endoscopic field of view. In this exact position, after the instrument is carefully retracted, one can see the most important landmark, the plica duodeni – a longitudinal fold that crosses the circular duodenal folds.

This fold corresponds to the intramural course of the common bile duct, leading the endoscopist to the papilla, which can be found at its end. According to the authors' observations, in the majority of cases the papilla is situated between the upper and the middle third of the descending duodenum at the medio-dorsal wall. While the longitudinal fold is a reliable guide to the endoscopist, the increasing pulsatory movements of the duodenal wall in the vicinity of the papilla may be of some help, too. They are caused by the gastroduodenal artery, which runs near the papilla.

The papilla of Vater appeares to the endoscopist as a raspberry-like protrusion, which is bounded cranially by a covering fold arising from the longitudinal fold (Fig. 13). In most cases observed by the authors, the papilla had a central pancreatic duct opening and a central common bile duct opening. Occasionally the orifice was eccentric. In these cases cannulation presented considerable difficulties. The endoscopic aspect of the normal papilla has a variety of forms.

Yet, in pathologic conditions, such as in cholelithiasis, with previous passage of calculi through the papilla, in benign or malign papillary stenoses, there is an even greater number of variations. Occasionally the papilla may be so flat and inconspicious that only the longitudinal folds may lead to its detection.

Cannulation should be performed in a close face-on view of the papilla, i.e. the papilla is in the center of the field of view (Fig. 14). Tangential cannulation is possible. However, as a rule, adequate filling of the duct system can only be achieved when the catheter cannulates the papilla at an angle of 90°.

The onset of peristalsis, which can be due to stretching of the stomach by the endoscope and which depends on the duration of the examination, can be suppressed by injection of spasmolytics. However, the periods of adequate duodenal ileus become shorter with increasing number of injections. The authors use Buscopan – 20 mg per transvenous injection – which instantly provides a good duodenal ileus. It lasts for a period of several minutes, depending on the dilatation of the duodenal wall, which is caused by insufflated air and the maneuvers of the instrument. Glucagon, which can be given transvenously – 1 mg per injection – has a longer lasting spasmolytic effect.

3.3.2 Roentgenology in ERPC

Injection of Contrast Medium and Roentgenologic Examination

After cannulation of the papilla, contrast material is injected into the pancreatic duct system. The duct of Wirsung is opacified as well as the side branches of first and second order. Opacification of the acinar

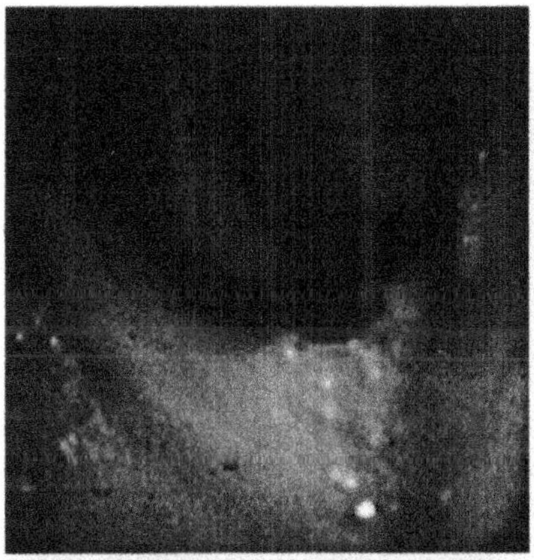

Fig. 8a

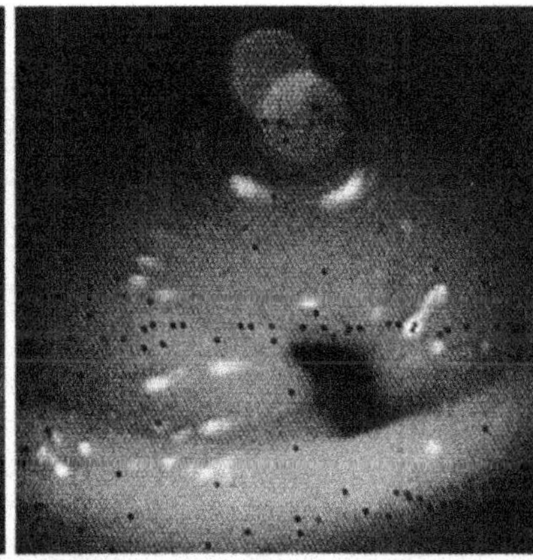

Fig. 9a

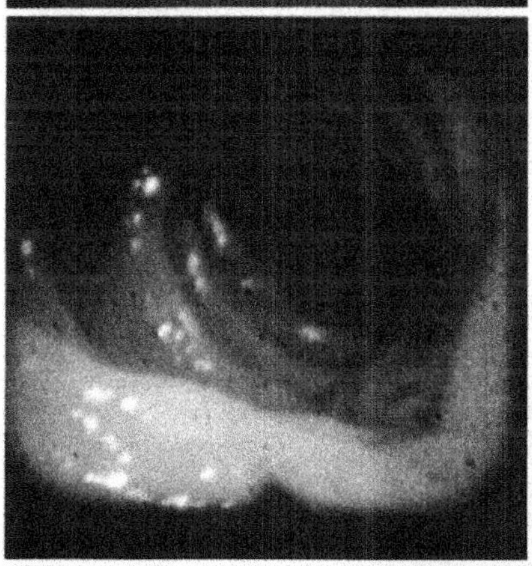

Fig. 11a

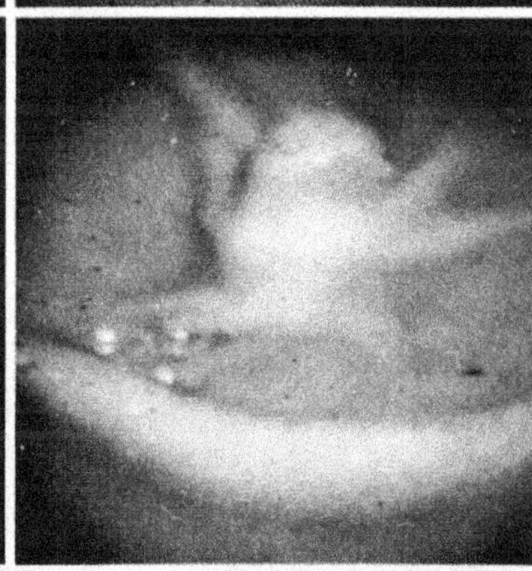

Fig. 13

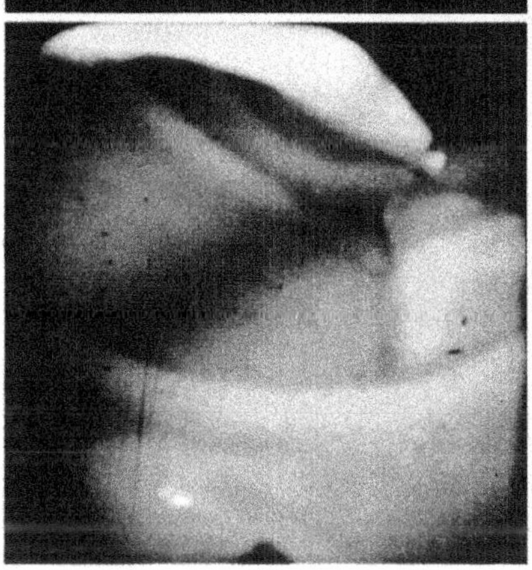

Fig. 14

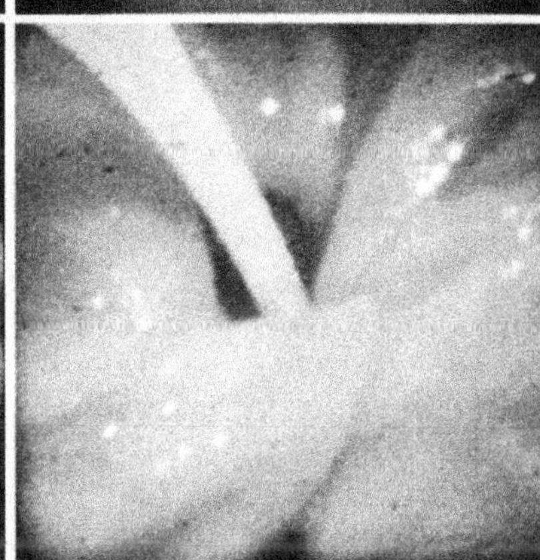

Fig. 15

Legends to Figs. 8a, 9a, and 11a see p. 16 and 18

Fig. 13. Endoscopic view of papilla of Vater. Raspberry-like papilla protrudes into duodenal lumen at oral end of plica longitudinalis duodeni. In lower sector of field of view a Kerckring's fold can be seen

Fig. 14. Endoscopic view of papilla of Vater and cannula immediately before cannulation of papilla

Fig. 15. Papilla is situated at margin of a deep duodenal diverticulum, cannula is introduced for better demonstration. One can recognize papilla as well as convergent Kerckring's folds ductal structure and the periacinar tissue should be avoided. In order to avoid such an "overfilling," the contrast material is injected under television fluoroscopic control. Consequently, television monitoring with high resolving power is indispensable. The attempt to standardize the injection pressure failed, since it is impossible to measure the actual pressure of the contrast medium when it passes from the catheter tip into the duct system. Experiments on resected specimen and on catheters showed a probable pressure of about 200 mg hg.

After the duct system has been filled, roentgenograms are made in lateral, in frontal, and if necessary, in further projections. When the duct system empties quickly, so that it is not possible to demonstrate it on roentgenograms after having changed the patient's position, cannulation and injection of dye should be repeated. ERPC films of 18 by 24 cm have proved favorable. As a rule, all segments of the duct systems can be documentated on films of these size. If necessary, spot films on special segments are made, especially for documentation of the motility and emptying function of the papilla.

3.4 Technical Difficulties in ERPC

The most frequent causes of difficulties in cannulation of the papilla are:

1. The abnormal site of the papilla at the border or at the bottom of a duodenal diverticulum (Fig. 15). According to the great number of varieties in duodenal diverticula, the site of the papilla in the diverticulum is quite variable. An intradiverticular papilla that is situated near the opening may present only minor technical problems, whereas the shape of the diverticulum becomes more decisive for successful cannulation the deeper the papilla is situated in the duodenum. If the diverticulum has a large opening and a wide neck, the papilla can be cannulated even if it is situated at the bottom. On the other hand, cannulation may fail in a papilla that is situated near the margin of the diverticulum when the opening is too narrow. Occasionally spasmolytics can be useful for flatening the duodenum and for widening its opening.

2. Papillary spasm: Spasm of the proper musculature of the orifice can considerably impede successful cannulation. In spite of correct positioning of the optic and the catheter, the latter cannot be advanced into the papilla. In these cases the spasm of the papilla may be a reaction to the contact with the catheter. The authors observed, that in such conditions, spasmolytics seem to relax the papillary muscle fibers so that cannulation may be possible at least for some minutes after intravenous injection. The same applies to the muscles of the prepapillary terminal duct systems of the pancreatic duct and of the common bile duct. Occasionally the nonopacified duct system can be filled after injection of spasmolytics.

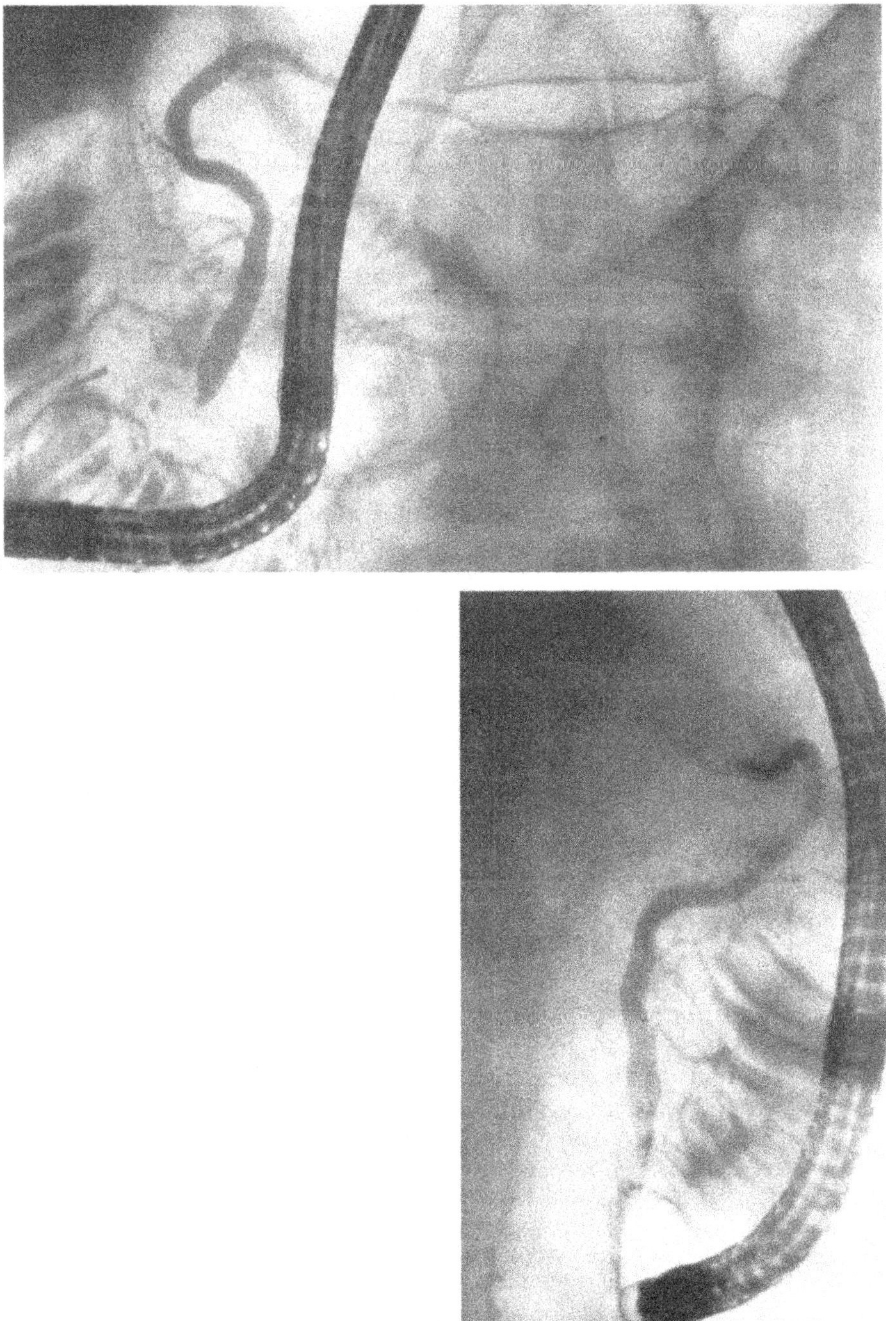

a

b

Fig. 16a and b. Cannulation of papilla and opacification of pancreatic duct system in patient with Billroth II stomach. Tip of instrument is in afferent loop. The instrument has already been straightened

3. Stenosis of the papilla, whether benign or malignant, can considerably impede successful cannulation. In benign stenoses the opening of the papilla can generally be seen and cannulated, but opacification of the duct system may not always be possible due to the narrowing of the orifice and the increased introductal pressure. However, in most malignant stenoses the examiner may already encounter endoscopic difficulties since the infiltrating tumor does not allow clear and safe delimitation of papillary and duodenal tissue. The orifice opens in the center of the ragged tumor protuberances, which are covered with secretion and show contact bleeding. In this condition cannulation may fail and diagnosis is established by biopsy (see Chapter 7.7).

4. Further difficulties include endoscopic problems, such as pyloric stenoses, postoperative adhesions with displacement of the duodenum and consecutive changes of the site of the papilla, as well as duodenal hyperperistalsis, which does not respond to spasmolytics.

5. Serious difficulties may arise in patients previously subjected to Billroth II surgery (Fig. 16a, b). If the anastomosis of the afferent loop is close to the cardia, it may be very difficult to obtain a face-on view of the papilla. The side-viewing optic is apparently not ideal, at least for the passage of the anastomosis. However, in inverted position of the instruments, endoscopy of the distal segments of the afferent loop is possible. After having turned the instrument clockwise, the experienced endoscopist can push deeper into the proximal segment of the afferent loop for cannulation of the papilla. Compared with the duration of the examination under normal conditions, ERPC is rather time-consuming in a patient with a Billroth II stomach. There is an additional risk, due to the fact that the tip of the instrument may glide into the cardia, since the anastomosis of the loop is in its immediate neighbourhood. Osnes and Miren report on an uncommonly high successful cannulation rate in Billroth II stomachs. In 17 of 20 patients that had previously been subjected to Billroth II surgery, endoscopy of the afferent loop with the Olympus JFB II duodenoscope could be performed. In 16 cases (80%) cannulation of the papilla was successful. Osnes and Miren developed and used a stiffening wire. After localization of the anastomosis of the afferent loop, the wire was introduced into the instrument channel. By means of this stiffening device, the endoscope could be pushed forward toward the papilla, which could be localized and cannulated after the wire had been removed. ERPC in a patient previously subjected to Billroth I surgery does not present any difficulties.

4. Indications, Contraindications, and Complications

4.1 Indications for ERPC

Since 1970 the indications for ERPC have been subject to considerable changes with increasing experience. In the beginning, when utmost precaution seemed to be advisable, the indications were strictly limited. In the course of time the relative safety of this examination and its diagnostic efficiency increased its frequency on a large scale. During this period, in the authors' case material, ERPC became a kind of screening method. However, with increasing experience, after the results had been compared and coordinated with other examinations of the pancreas, well-defined indications could be established. Consequently, the rate of pathologic findings increased considerably in the authors' material.

With regard to the contraindications, the following indications for ERPC seem to be justified:

1. The clinically substantiated suspicion of a lesion of the excretory pancreatic system, especially:
   a) Suspicion of chronic pancreatitis or chronic relapsing pancreatitis for checking of the drainage function
   b) Suspicion of sequelae secondary to pancreatitis such as necrosis with sequestration and formation of a pseudocyst
   c) Suspicion of pancreatic carcinoma
2. Suspicion of benign or malignant papillary stenosis
3. Suspicion of extrahepatic cholostasis when transvenous cholangiography fails, particularly in:
   a) Obstructive jaundice of unknown origin
   b) In cases of nonopacification of the gallbladder in the transvenous cholangiogram when the extrahepatic ducts are well-visualized
4. Uncleared upper abdominal pain in patients that have been previously subjected to cholecystectomy or to cholangiodigestive anastomosis.

4.2 Contraindications

Inoperability or nonconsent of the patient is a general contraindication, otherwise, in case of considerable retention of juice or filling of a necrotic cavity, relieving surgical intervention cannot be performed for prevention of infection.

Special contraindications:
1. Acute pancreatitis.
2. The true pancreatic cyst.
3. Necrotic or postnecrotic cavities when the diagnosis has been sufficiently established by other methods. If reliable diagnosis cannot be established by conventional diagnostic methods, the authors perform preoperative ERPC for demonstration and localization of the cavity.
4. Acute purulent cholangitis. Esophageal varices are not considered an absolute contraindication, provided that the examination does not take much time and that gross motion of the instrument are avoided.

4.3 Hazards, Complications, and Treatment

Hazards, complications, and the need for surgical intervention are in close relation to indications and contraindications of ERPC. Considerable changes of the pancreatic duct system that necessitate relieving surgical intervention can be found in ERPC, even in patients with rather inconspicuous clinical findings and functional tests. Consequently, those changes cannot always be foreseen. Hence, the patient's operability and consent must always be cleared before ERPC can be performed. In the advanced stage of chronic pancreatitis the danger lies in the fact that emptying of contrast material is occasionally delayed. The dye can be kept back in necrotic cavities and pseudocysts giving rise to infection. In those cases, infection of the retained fluid can only be avoided if the obstruction is relieved by surgical intervention within 24 h. The same problems may be encountered in obstructive jaundice, or in advanced extrahepatic cholostasis of different origin such as calculi in the bile ducts, iatrogenic stenoses, tumor encasement of the bile ducts due to pancreatic carcinoma, primary extrahepatic carcinoma of the bile ducts, benign or malignant papillary stenoses, and further obstructive lesions, such as pancreatic pseudocysts or enlarged lymph nodes. The emptying time, controlled by television monitoring, is decisive for the timing of surgery. As to the pancreatic duct, the emptying time should not exceed much more than 10 min with regard to the pathomorphologic changes. The contrast material in the bile ducts should be considerably diluted 20 min after the last injection.

In addition to surgical intervention in extrahepatic cholostasis, antibiotics should be administered preoperatively. Otherwise, if surgical intervention is not performed, the risk of complications with fatal outcome is considerably high in cases of pancreatic necrosis of pseudocysts with marked retention of pancreatic juice or bile.

Independent of one another, Amann (1973), Classen (1973), and Cotten (1973), reported on fatal hazards in ERPC in patients with pseudocysts. Of 1850 examinations the authors observed two cases with fatal complications after ERPC. These two patients presenting pancreatic tumor encasement of the common bile duct and pseudocyst, respectively, were not operated upon after ERPC. Thus, in the authors' case material, the fatal complication rate amounts to 0.1%.

The problem of elevation of serum lipase secondary to ERPC has been studied by two independent teams. The results of the report of Grimmel et al. (1974) are largely identical with those found by Bornschein et al. (1974). In the authors' case material, a significant increase of activity up to 6,380 U/l·min was found in 36 of 46 cases (Fig. 17). This elevation of lipase was not accompanied by clinical symptoms. Of this group, 13 patients had slightly elevated serum lipase levels. The average increase of lipase was not higher in these patients than in the cases of normal initial lipase levels. All patients showed a decreasing lipase activity 24 h after ERPC. In 20 of the 36 patients that had shown an increase of activity, the lipase levels had normalized within 48 h. All 13 patients with initially increased lipase activity were found in the next group of 16 patients, that showed increased activity 48 h after ERPC. In this group 11 patients had changes secondary to chronic

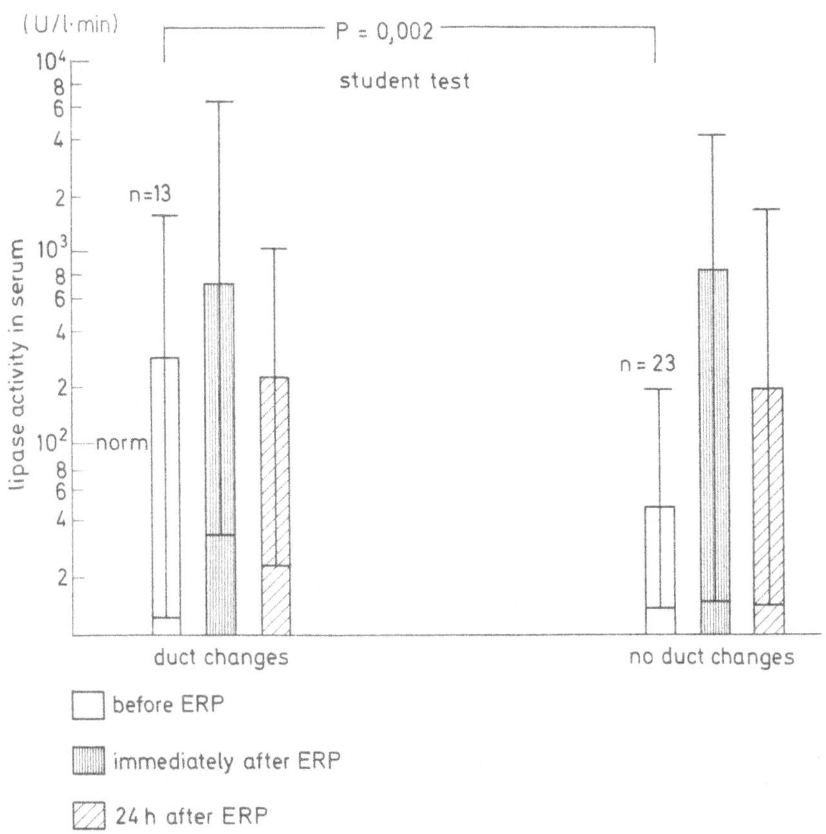

Fig. 17. Lipase activity in serum. Diagram shows that almost inevitable increase in lipase activity secondary to ERPC is almost same in normal and pathologically changed duct systems. (From Bornschein et al., 1974)

pancreatitis, with or without pancreatic necrosis, one had dysontogenetic cysts, and two pancreatic carcinomas. Two patients presented with a normal duct system; the clinical signs were compatible with acute or chronic hepatitis.

A comparative study shows that there is no statistically relevant difference in the rate of elevation and decrease in serum lipase activity after ERPC in normal and pathologic duct systems with the exception of those cases that presented with an increased average level of serum lipase prior to ERPC (Fig. 18).

There is, however, a significant relation between the filling degree and the elevation of lipase activity (Fig. 19). In all cases with opacification of acinar or periacinar tissue, an obvious elevation of lipase activity could be observed. Especially the 24 h values are statistically significant. Grimmel et al. (1974) report similar results. These authors observed the elevation of lipase activity in one of four patients with opacification of the pancreatic main duct and its side branches, in seven of eight patients with opacification of the side branches of first and second order, and in all patients with acinar opacification. Hence, "overfilling" with acinar opacification should be strictly avoided. On the other hand, Galvan and Klotz (1972) report on acute pancreatitis secondary to ERPC in cases in which only a few centimeters of the main duct had been opacified.

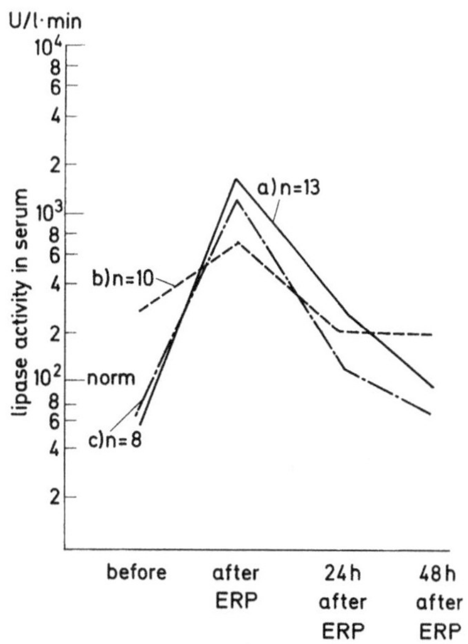

Fig. 18. Diagram from same publication as shown in Fig. 17. Serum lipase activity after ERPC has dropped to normal about 48 h after examination. Already 24 h later level drops distinctly. Here again there is no substantial difference in serum lipase activity between normal and pathologically changed duct system

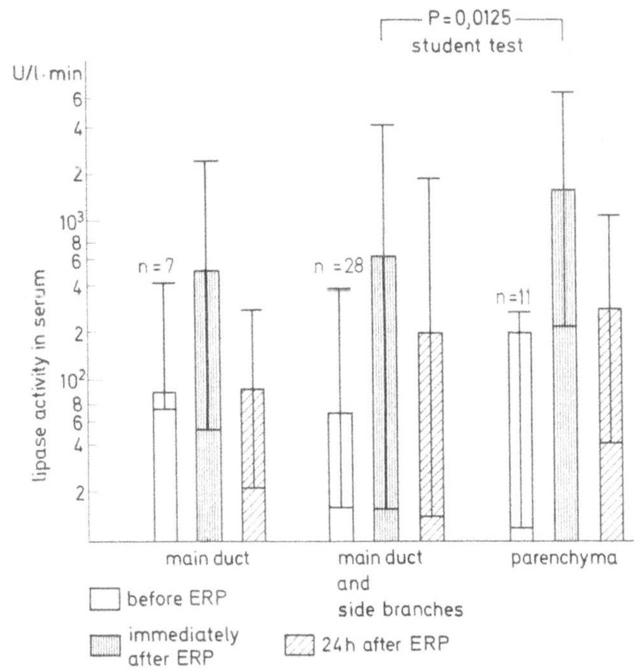

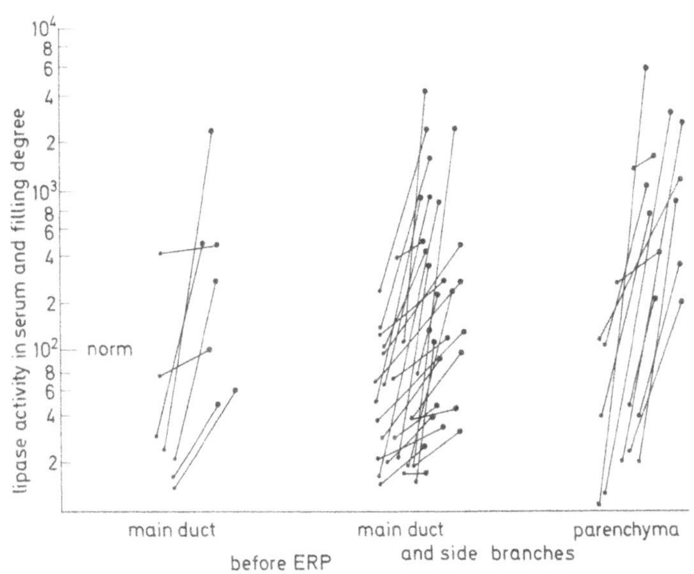

Fig. 19. Diagram from same publication mentioned above. Significant increase in serum lipase activity in cases with acinar and periacinar opacification compared with cases showing only opacification of main duct and of side branches or of main duct alone

However, the authors believe that the risk of provoking acute pancreatitis by ERPC is rather small. Nevertheless, acute inflammation after ERPC cannot be definitely prevented. Consequently the indication for ERPC should be restricted to clinically well-defined cases. In case of doubt, considering the pros (the high diagnostic efficiency) and the cons (the small complication rate) it may be better to perform ERPC than to put up with an incomplete or false diagnosis.

5. The Normal Retrograde Pancreaticogram

Numerous anatomical studies and peroperative pancreaticographies provide us a good knowledge of the normal aspect of the pancreatic duct system as well as of its main variants. Yet, in endoscopic retrograde pancreaticography, there are some particularities that should be considered. For only the exact knowledge of the normal retrograde pancreaticogram and its variants allow us to assess pathologic changes.

5.1 Site of the Papilla of Vater

The characteristic anatomical features of the papilla and the descending duodenum may lead the experienced endoscopist to its localization in the descending duodenum. Yet, it may be of some use for the learner to know the most common site of the papilla in the descending part of the duodenum. For this purpose the pathologist's studies are of little use, because in the resected specimen the topographic situation of the papilla differs by far from that in the living patient. This accounts for the fact, that, as to the site of the papilla, the findings made by the endoscopists are in some contradiction to the report by Becker (1973), who found the papilla in 73% in the lower third of the second duodenum and in 18% in the intermediate third. Most authors localize the papilla of Vater in the upper third of the second duodenum. In a smaller percentage the papilla was found in the upper and in the intermediate third [Cotton (1972), Jeanpierre (1971), Weiss et al. (1973)]. In the authors' material the papilla was found in the upper third in 20%, in the intermediate third in 70% and in 10% in the lower third of the descending duodenum. Only Classen et al. (1973) localized the papilla 8 times (16%) in the upper third, 27 times (50%) in the intermediate third, and 15 times (30%) in the lower third out of 50 patients.

5.2 The Anatomy of the Papilla of Vater

The anatomical structure of the papilla, the common or separate outlet of the bile duct or of the pancreatic duct, the existence of an ampulla of Vater, as well as the fine structure of the mucosa folds at the level of the sphincter of Oddi may be of decisive importance for cannulation of the papilla and for simultaneous filling of the bile duct. According to Sterling's studies, the pancreatic main duct and the common

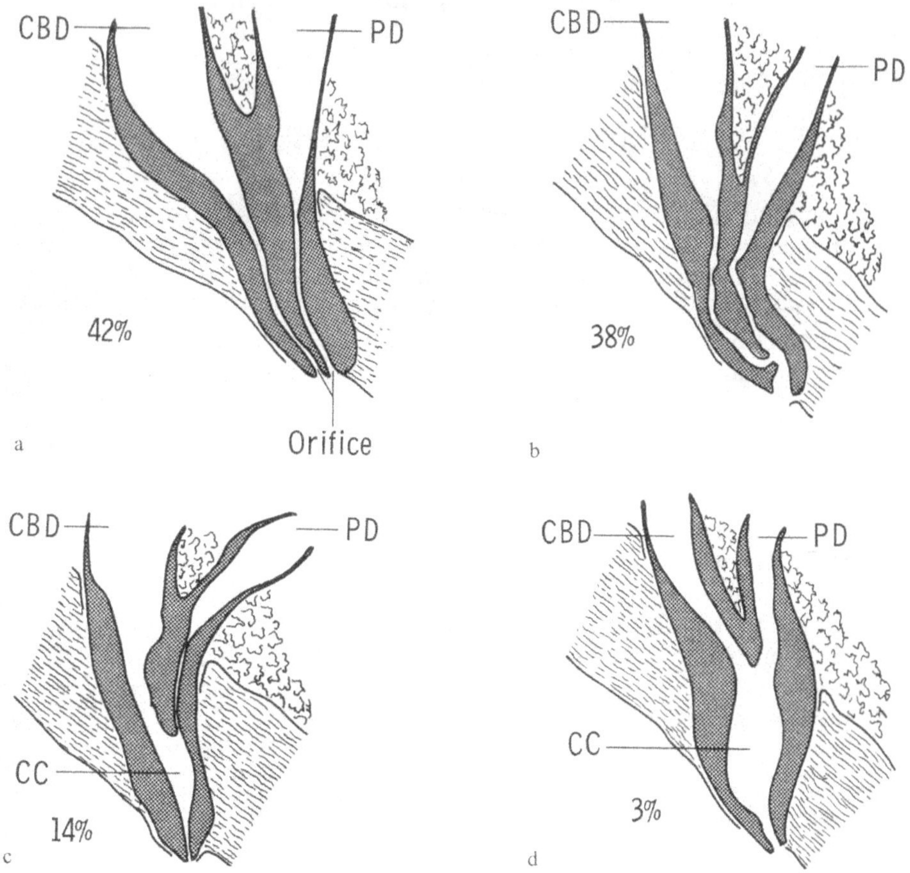

Fig. 20a–d. Anatomic structure of papilla of Vater (According to Sterling)

bile duct form, respectively, a common duct and an ampullae of Vater in 55% (Fig. 20b–d). Yet, in 38% this common duct is only a few millimeters long whereas ampullae of various sizes can be found in 17%. In 42% the common bile duct and the pancreatic duct open separately into the papilla (Fig. 20a). This means that after successful cannulation of the pancreatic main duct, which as a rule, is filled first in almost half of all cases, cannulation must be repeated in order to find the opening of the bile duct. Furthermore, the anatomical situation as shown in Figure 20b may explain that, due to the slight pressure with which the catheter is introduced, it can push into the tissue protuberance which lies in the front of the common bile duct and consequently prevent filling of the duct in 38%. Out of 66 specimens, the authors found in only 3 cases (4.5%) a small tissue bridge between the pancreatic duct and the bile duct. These findings may explain the fact, that, according to the reports of all authors, the pancreatic duct is cannulated in a higher percentage than the common bile

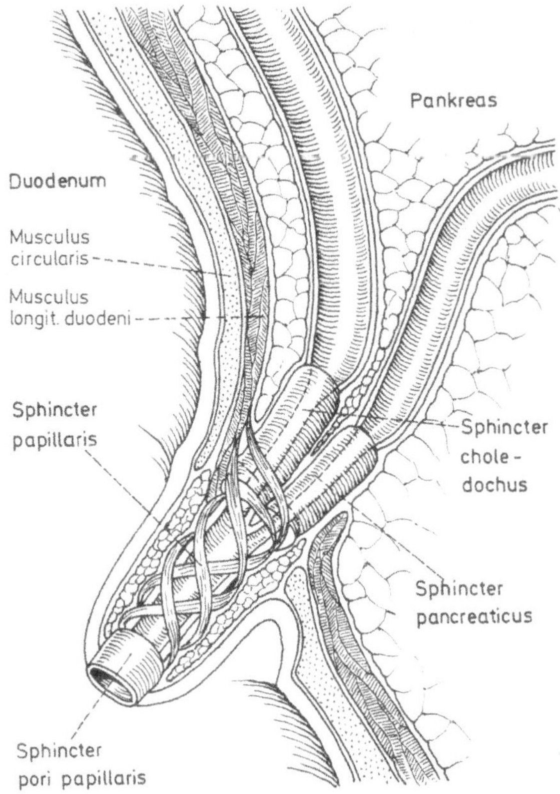

Fig. 21. Anatomic structure of sphincter muscles of papilla. (According to Hentschel)

duct, regardless of the kind of cannulation, whether by means of balloon-catheter, peroperative cannulation or endoscopic cannulation. Furthermore, the anatomical structure may explain why sometimes one can succeed in filling the bile duct after the pancreatic duct has already been filled by slow retraction of the catheter and simultaneous injection of contrast material. Another cause for the lower rate of successful filling of the bile ducts may be the fact that there may be two separate sphincter muscles around the orifice of the bile duct and the pancreatic duct (Fig. 21). Thus, the stronger sphincter of the bile duct may contract more closely than the less efficient sphincter of the pancreatic duct when the papilla is irritated during cannulation.

5.3 Main Duct and Side Branches of the Pancreas

The pancreatic duct system is arranged on the main channel principle. The main channel is the duct of Wirsung or the duct of Santorini.

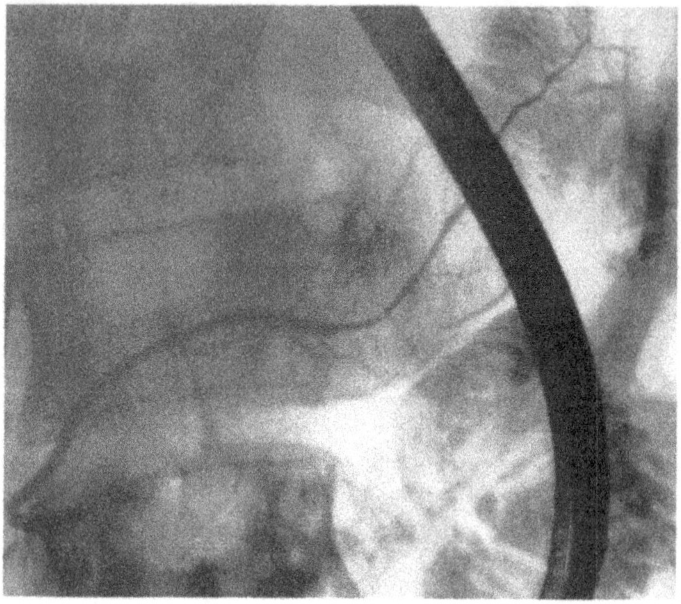

Fig. 22. Normal pancreatic duct system with pancreatic main duct (Wirsung's duct and numerous rami pancreatici)

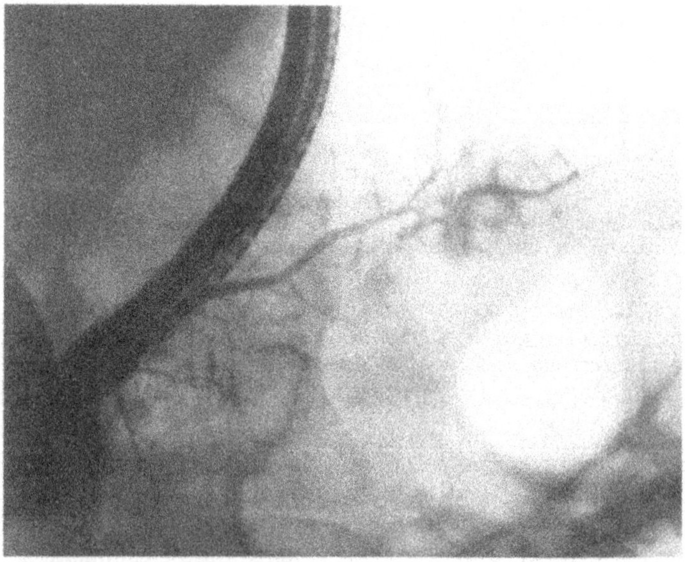

Fig. 23. Cephalad prominent part of pancreatic body, which is drained by large ramus with several ductuli. Incomplete acinar opacification

In the head of the gland, the duct of Wirsung runs upward in a high angle. In the isthmus it changes its direction running more horizontally, and in the tail its course is again directed upward laterally (Fig. 22).

Here it ends in a fine terminal network of branches, or in 10% it bifurcates into small branches, the ramus caudae superior and inferior. The upper and lower parts of the gland are drained by 15–30 side branches, the rami pancreatici superiores and inferiores, respectively, which open into the duct of Wirsung. In the majority of cases only a small number of these rami are opacified in retrograde pancreaticography. Sometimes one of those branches drains a somewhat prominent segment of the gland by means of several side branches. We defined them, as well as the other side branches of the rami as ductuli. If such a larger ramus empties into the head of the gland above or below the duct of Wirsung, they are called ramus corporis superior, ramus corporis inferior, respectively (Fig. 23). In retrograde pancreaticography, such a ramus is often filled, even if only a small number of smaller rami are opacified. Localized duplication of the pancreatic main duct has been found to be a very rare anomaly (Fig. 59). In the two cases observed by the authors, there was an abscess in the vicinity of the duplication of the duct.

Small circular or oval cysts at the terminal segments of the rami pancreatici are a very rare malformation (Fig. 24). If they do not pass beyond the confines of the gland or cause compression, they are mere accessory findings of no clinical interest.

The rami are divided into further branches, the so-called ductuli, which are yet less frequently opacified in ERPC. The ductuli themselves are divided into canaliculi (Fig. 25b). They are almost never demonstrated in retrograde pancreaticography. Not all of the side branches of the pancreatic main duct join the duct of Wirsung in the downstream direction. Yet, the pattern of the course of the side branches of the

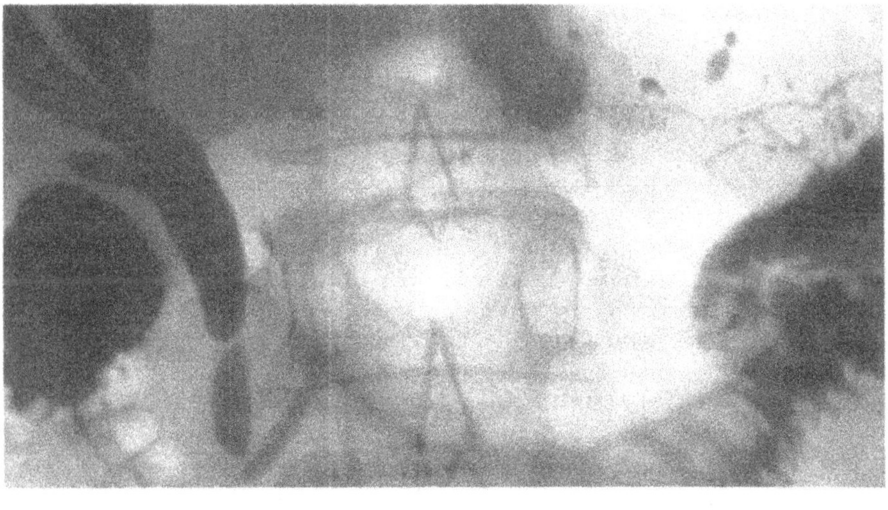

Fig. 24. Multiple small cysts at terminal segments of the rami pancreatici. Malformation

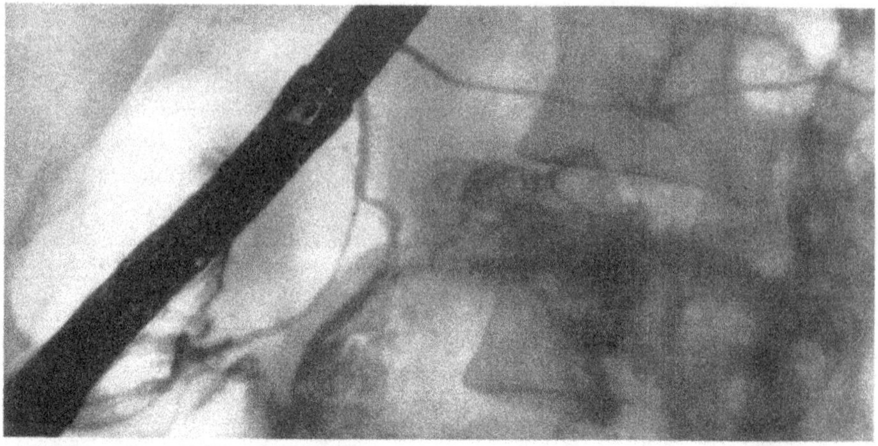

a

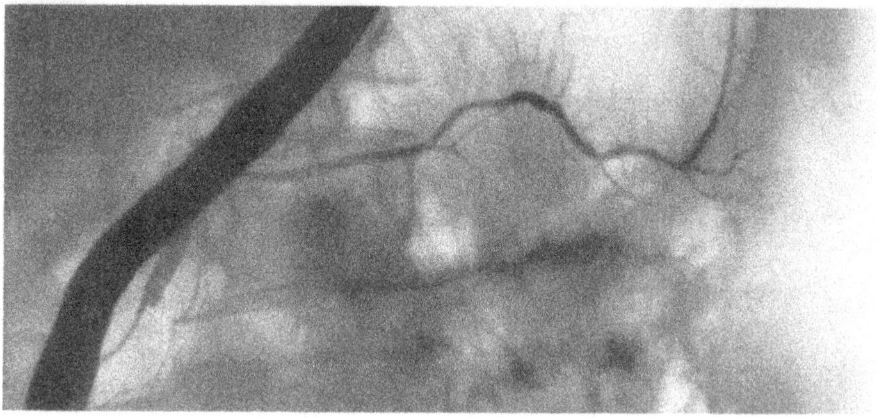

b

Fig. 25a and b. Santorini's duct running above (a) and below (b) duct of Wirsung with own orifice on minor papilla

duct of Santorini is by far less regular. One can find even a large side branch joining the duct of Santorini at a sharp angle and in the upstream direction. Thus, neither the angle nor its caliber can give sufficient information about the actual flow of the pancreatic juice and consequently about the existence of a separate opening into the duodenum. In 64 resected specimens the authors found the duct of Santorini running above the main duct in 34 (53%) (Fig. 25a) and below the pancreatic main duct in 30 (47%) (Fig. 25b). Here (according to the findings of Gualdi and Messe, 1959, in 76%) it takes up a major side branch, the ramus capitis inferior. This branch drains the largest part of the pancreatic head. In 41% the ramus capitis inferior (Fig. 26) does not join the duct of Santorini but opens into the duct of Wirsung (Gualdi and Messe) (Fig. 27). If the duct of Santorini is situated below the duct of Wirsung, the ramus capitis runs to the upper part of the head. In such a case it may be best to define it

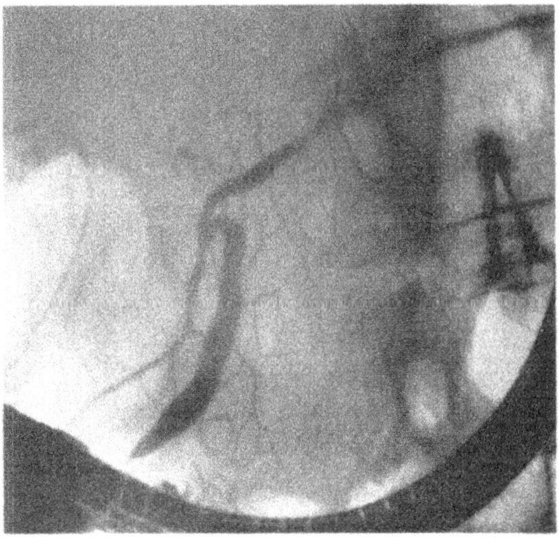

Fig. 26. Santorini's duct with several rami capitis inferiores, which drain head of gland

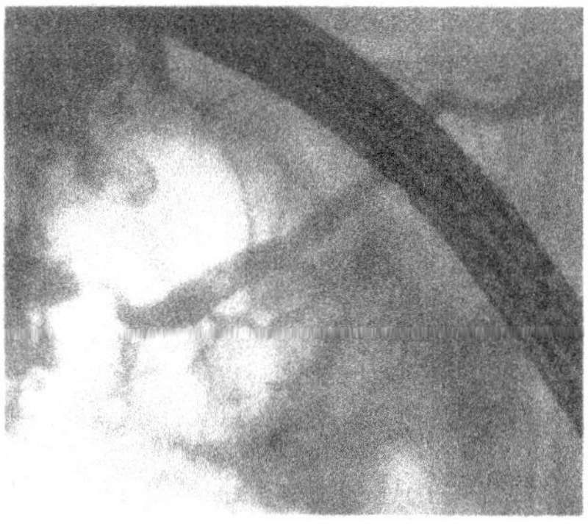

Fig. 27. Ramus capitis inferior joins Wirsung's duct

as ramus capitis superior. According to Rienhoff and Lewis (1934) in 24–30% of all cases, the duct of Santorini communicates with the duct of Wirsung. In only 1 of 71 resected specimens did the authors not find any major communications between the two main ducts. They could only find anastomoses via the smallest canaliculi. Of the authors' ERPC case material, opacification of only the duct of Santorini and some of its side branches without opacification of the duct of Wirsung could be observed in 65 cases (Figs. 28a, b, c). The knowledge of these anatomical variants is of practical importance as they should not be mistaken for partial obstruction of the duct system. In about 20% of all cases the duct of Santorini is obliterated (Opie, 1927; Schirmer), in 1–2% it had not developed at all (Schirmer).

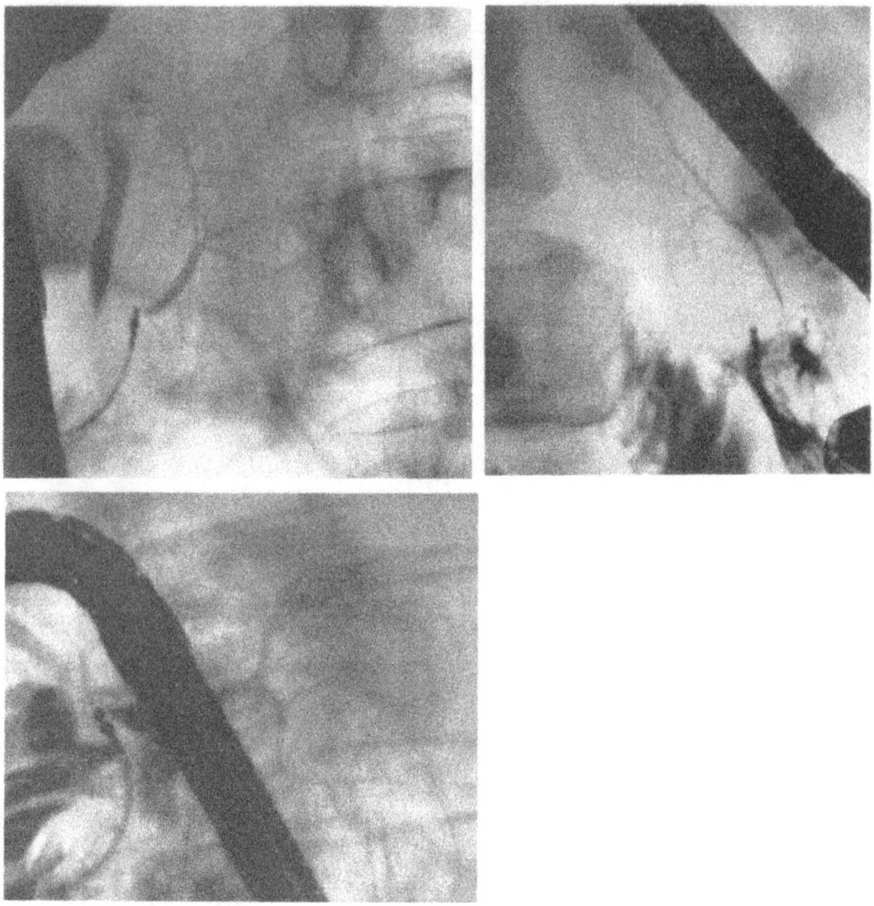

Fig. 28a–c. Selective demonstration of Santorini's duct, which opens into duodenum on papilla of Vater. Head of pancreas is exclusively drained by Santorini's duct. Normal aspect of common bile duct

5.4 Width of the Pancreatic Main Duct

The width of the main duct is of special importance for the assessment of several pathologic conditions. It has been examined in resected specimens and in retrograde pancreaticographies by numerous authors. Of 50 anatomical specimens, the authors found an average width of 3–4 mm at the largest segment of the duct, ranging between 1–6 mm (Anacker, 1961). In 1959 Birnstingl found a somewhat larger average width of 4.1 mm with a range of 1.8–9.2 mm. Of 100 retrograde pancreaticographies, the authors found in 1963 an average width of 2–3 mm of the duct of Wirsung with a range of 1–6 mm. This difference may be explained by the fact that in the anatomical specimen the duct

Fig. 29. Relative width of Wirsung's duct (duct width/vertebra/height ratio in different age groups)

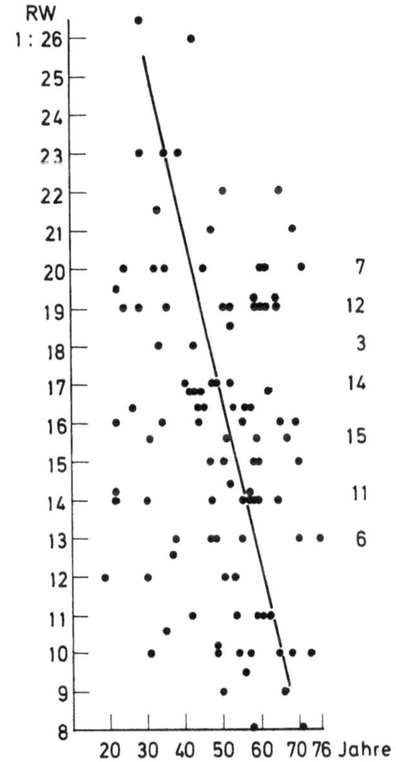

may have been more completely filled than in endoscopic pancreaticograms, in which the lumen may not have always been completely filled with contrast material. As in endoscopic retrograde pancreaticography, different factors depending on the condition of the examination (increased distance between object and film) may falsify radiologic measurements of the lumen. It may be useful to set the width of the duct in relation to the height of the neighboring vertebral body (Fig. 29). In 100 ERPCs the average ratio ranges between 1:14 and 1:19 (Fig. 34).

Since the lumen of the duct of Wirsung decreases from the head to the tail, it would be more correct to assess the width of three different segments. Classen et al. (1973) studied the average width of the duct in 40 cases. They found an average width of 4–5 mm with a range of 2–7 mm in 70% of their case material. In the body in 75% of their cases, the average width was 3–3.5 mm with a range of 1.5 and 5 mm. In the tail of the gland the majority of the ducts presented an average width of 2–3 mm with a range of 1–3 mm. The caliber of the side branches (rami pancreatici) averages 0.2 mm. They are 1–2 cm long. In view of the enormous range that has been found by all authors, the assessments of the width of the duct as to its pathologic relevance may not be very efficient in the isolated case. Fortunately, the majority of pathologic conditions of the pancreas that are associated with widening of the ducts presents further symptoms, so that when making a roentgenologic diagnosis, one is not exclusively dependent upon the symptom of ectasia.

Ectasia can be defined, too, as a loss of the normal tapering form of the main ducts, which normally decreases from the head to the tail. As in papillary stenosis the pancreatic duct or the common bile duct or both duct systems can be dilated. It may be of some use to know the relationship of the normal caliber of the pancreatic duct to that of the common bile duct. The authors found a ratio of 1–2 i.e., the common bile duct is generally twice as wide as the pancreatic duct.

In studies on 45 male and 45 female patients the authors could show that in normal cases the caliber of the pancreatic duct seems to be independent of the patient's sex.

5.5 Different Types and Variations of the Orifice

The frequency of the opening of the pancreatic main duct at the major papilla, as well as the frequency of the common orifice of the pancreatic duct, and of the bile duct is of special importance in ERPC. Of 500 cases, the authors found in 95.5% the orifice of the duct of Wirsung situated on the papilla of Vater. In only 3 cases (4.5%) the duct of Santorini opened on the major papilla. In studies on resected specimens Gualdi and Messe (1959) found a considerably higher incidence of this latter variation, which they could observe in 38%. These contradictory results may be due to differing identification of the ducts.

The variations and combinations of the openings of the common bile duct, the duct of Wirsung, and duct of Santorini are of special importance for ERPC as well as for surgical intervention. The authors' studies on 66 resected specimens showed that in 56 cases (85%) the duct of Wirsung and the common bile duct have a common orifice. In 9 cases (13.5%) the pancreatic main duct opened independently of the common bile duct at the major papilla (Anacker, 1967). The common orifice was found in 75% by Westphal (1936). Kleitsch (1955) found a common orifice in 90% of 33 cases; Hughes and Kernutt (1954) found a common orifice in all 26 of their cases. Theoretically, the common bile duct as well as the pancreatic duct could be filled by cannulation of the papilla in 85–90%. The intervening circumstances that may prevent simultaneous filling of the two duct systems have already been mentioned. In view of the fact that the number of orifices of the two duct systems are of decisive importance for ERPC and for surgical intervention, it may be useful to clarify three different types of openings (Fig. 30):

1. A single opening.

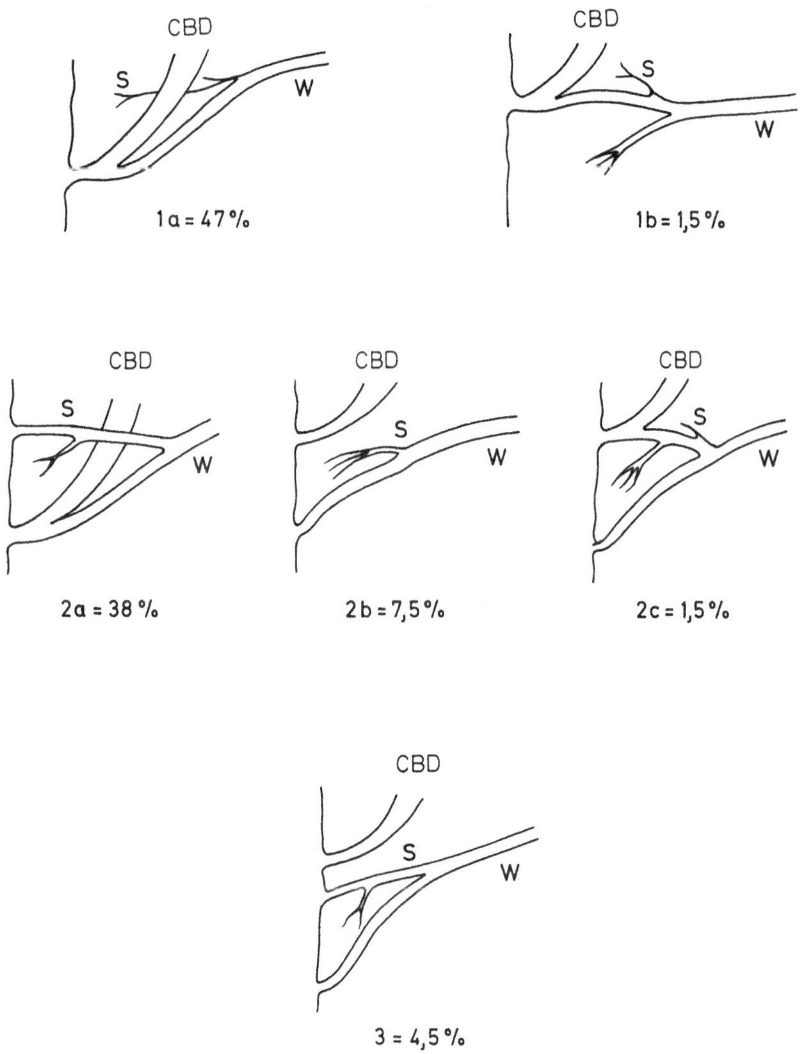

Fig. 30. Different types of openings of Wirsung's duct and common bile duct

a) The common bile duct and the duct of Wirsung have a common orifice. There is complete absence of the duct of Santorini or the latter may not have an opening of its own. The authors found this type in 31 cases (46%) of 66 anatomical specimens. Kleitsch (1955) reported on 70% from his case material, Schirmer found this type in 53%, Fritsch in 67%, Naatanen in 67%, Nuboer in 81%, and Schmieden and Sebening report on 20 cases of 35 specimens.

b) There is a common opening of the bile duct and the duct of Santorini. The duct of Wirsung has no orifice of its our. Out of 66

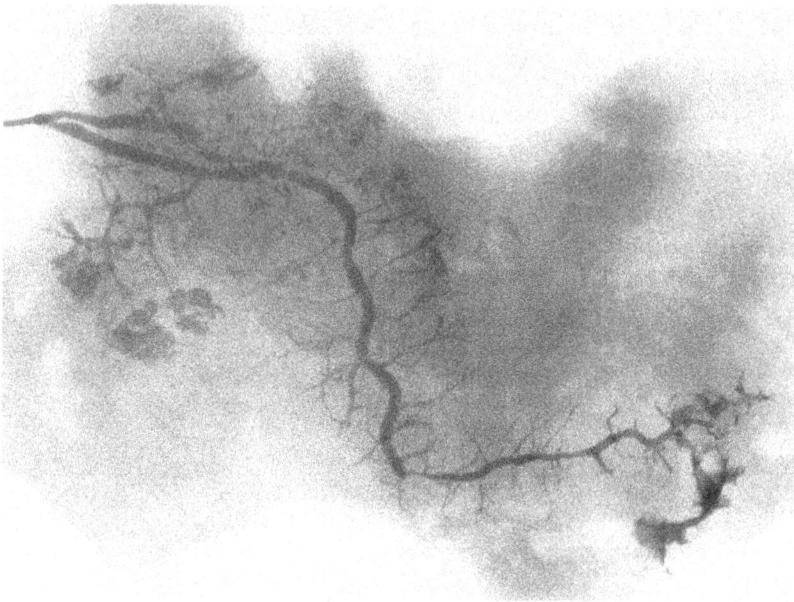

Fig. 31. Filling of pancreatic duct system of resected specimen with contrast material. Stenosis of Wirsung's duct between body and tail without prestenotic dilatation. Patient had died on acute hemorrhagic pancreatic necrosis

anatomical specimens the authors found this variation in only 1 case (1.5%).

2. Two openings.

a) There is a common opening of the bile duct and the duct of Wirsung on the major papilla. The duct of Santorini has a special opening on the minor papilla, which is generally situated orally to the papilla of Vater. The authors observed this anatomical variant in 25 cases (38%), Gualdi and Messe (1959) in 38%, Kleitsch (1955) in 60%.

b) There are separate openings of the common bile duct and the duct of Wirsung. There is no orifice of the duct of Santorini. The authors found this anatomical variant in 5 cases (7.5%). In these cases the duct of Wirsung and the common bile duct may open on the major or on the minor papilla.

c) The following anatomical variant is very rare: There is, mostly on the papilla of Vater, a common opening of the bile duct and the duct of Santorini, while the duct of Wirsung has a separate orifice at the minor papilla. The authors found this anatomical variant in only 1 specimen (1.5%). It may be of some use for ERPC to know that if the duct of Santorini has a separate opening into the duodenum, it generally communicates with the duct of Wirsung. It is rarely separat-

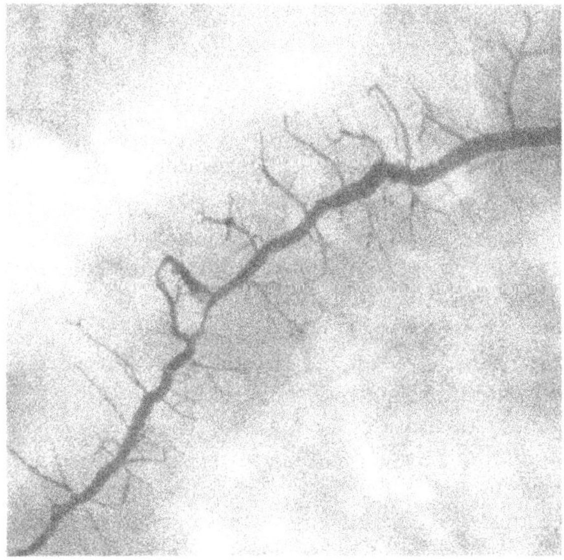

Fig. 32. Postmortem pancreaticogram. Stenosis of Wirsung's duct between body and tail. Stenosis is bridged by collateral duct. Slight escape of contrast medium from this collateral duct. Acute hemorrhagic pancreatic necrosis with clinical and pathologic signs and symptoms

ed from the remaining duct system. The authors observed such separate duct systems in 3 cases out of 500 examinations.

3. Three openings.

There are separate openings of the bile duct, the duct of Wirsung, and the duct of Santorini. The authors observed this condition in 3 (4.5%) out of 66 anatomical specimens. Out of the authors' case material only 1 case with an opening of the duct of Wirsung and the bile duct into a duodenal diverticulum was observed. In view of the technical difficulties in ERPC this finding may be of some importance. In the normal pancreas, circumscribed stenoses of the duct of Wirsung do exist. Of 63 anatomical specimens, the authors found 1 case of annular stenosis (1967), which obviously did not obstruct the normal flow of secretion since there was no prestenotic dilatation. In 3 cases the authors found 5–8-mm-long stenoses at the junction of the body and the tail (Fig. 31). Two of these cases were pancreatic necroses with fatal outcome. In one case the stenosis was bridged by a bypassing anastomosis (Fig. 31). A side branch of this bypassing duct was perforated.

Histologic examinations showed changes secondary to acute hemorrhagic pancreatic necrosis in this area. As there is no symptom of acute pancreatitis in the remaining part of the gland, the question arises whether the changes of the duct mentioned above and the perforation of the side branch might be considered as the releasing factor of the localized hemorrhagic pancreatic necrosis (Fig. 59). The authors observed a similar case in ERPC.

5.6 The Normal Emptying Process of the Pancreatic Duct

The emptying process of the pancreatic main duct is similar to that of the common bile duct. The different phases that can be observed are closely dependent on the anatomical structure of the major papilla. Apart from the sphincter pori papillaris, the common sphincter of the two duct systems, the common bile duct as well as the pancreatic duct each have their own sphincter muscle (Fig. 21). On principle, this structure implies a separate function of each sphincter and consequently separate emptying of bile and pancreatic juice, independent of one another. This can actually be observed in some rare cases. Separate emptying may be favored by the fact that, according to Harm's findings and the authors' examinations on retrograde pancreaticographies, the intraductal pancreatic pressure is generally higher than the pressure in the bile duct, since the average pancreatic duct pressure amounts to 22.2 cm of water. On the other hand, the presence of sphincter muscles may explain, that evacuation is actively controled by the sphincter muscle as soon as the pressure in the duct has reached a certain amount. This can easily be demonstrated when the pancreatic duct is faintly opacified and the patient is brought in upright position, so that contrast material accumulates in the prepapillary segment of the duct. Then, with increasing intraductal pressure, the emptying phase begins. One can differentiate three phases:

1. The emptying phase.

Under television monitoring the emptying phase is easily identified by an ejection of contrast material. On a roentgenogram it is marked by a small filiform line of contrast material, continuing the direction of the tapered end of the pancreatic duct into the duodenum (Fig. 33 D). This contrast line may take a rectilinear, a hooked, or a spiral course in the papillary segment of the pancreatic duct, as well as of the bile duct. These patterns are determinated by the action of muscle fibers of longitudinal or helical arrangement and does not indicate pathology. Generally the emptying phase lasts only for a few seconds.

2. The contraction phase.

The sphincter muscle contracts and pushes the dye back into the duct. On the film the opacified pancreatic duct and bile duct seem to end several milimeters to 1 cm away from the duodenal wall. Their end can be tapered, club-shaped or convex (Fig. 33a). The concave shape, as it can be observed at the distal bile duct during a marked contraction, cannot be found at the pancreatic duct. This may be due to the less developed muscular strength of its sphincter. The duration of the contraction phase always corresponds to that of the emptying phase, which differs from one case to another.

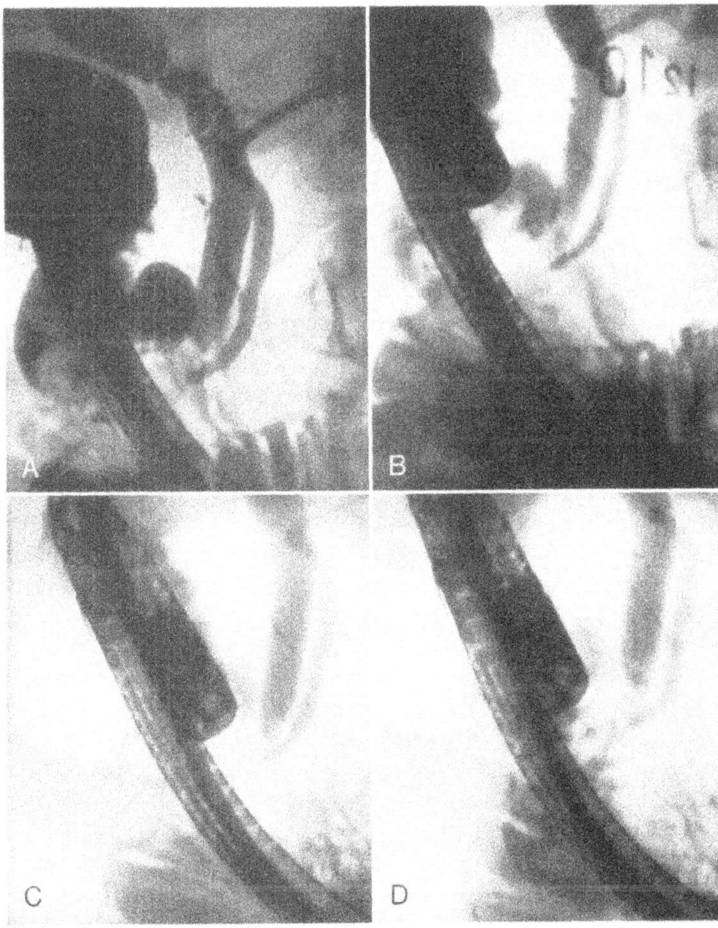

Fig. 33A–D. Motion study of papilla. Emptying phase (*D*). Contrast material empties from Wirsung's duct and common bile duct into duodenum. During contraction phase (*A*) contrast material is kept back by papillary muscles. In recreation phase (*B*) papillary muscles relax (*C*) Tapered shape of intrapapillary segment

3. The recreation phase.

The opacified area in the pancreatic duct, as well as the bile duct end in a pencil-like tapered shape near the duodenal wall (Fig. 33b). According to the decrease of pressure in an advanced emptying process, the number and duration of the recreation phases increases. It goes without saying, that complete emptying depends on the entire quantity of the injected contrast material, i.e., on the total of the lumina of the ducts. Generally the emptying process takes 2–7 min. In the majority of the cases the pancreatic duct and the bile duct empty simultaneously in a synchronous sequence of the different phases. Of 270 examinations the authors observed only 2 cases presenting independent, alternating emptying phases of the bile duct and the pancreatic duct respectively (Anacker et al., 1973). In the case of a separate orifice of the duct of Santorini at the minor papilla, the emptying process seems to follow a rhythmic succession of opening and closing of the minor papilla. The authors could find this kind of emptying phase in 5 cases. However, the minuteness of the structures do not allow for a definitive statement.

5.7 Transpapillary Pressure Measurement in the Pancreatic Duct and the Common Bile Duct

When deep cannulation of the two duct systems was revealed to be a relatively safe procedure, studies on selective pressure measurement were made on a large scale. Chronic inflammatory and malignant lesions were expected to cause pathologic changes of intraductal pressure, either by retention of pancreatic juice or bile or by reduced secretion.

The authors have developed a simple and efficient method for pressure measurement in the two duct systems. The first preliminary study was made on the normal physiologic and the average basic pressure in the pancreatic duct and the common bile duct in relatively large case material.

Studies on pressure measurements in animals were made first by Henry and Wollheim in 1876. These authors studied the intraductal pressure of the pancreatic main duct of narcotized rabbits. They found a pressure of 21.9–22.5 cm of water. In 1909 Herring and Simpson found a pressure of 24.0–31.8 cm of water in three narcotized dogs after stimulation of secretion by duodenal extract. These pressures correspond to an average pressure of 31.3 cm of water. In the common bile duct an average pressure of 30 cm of water was recorded.

In order to eliminate the effect of anesthesia, Harms, in 1924, studied secretion of the pancreatic and the biliary duct system under physiologic conditions. The experiments were carried out on five dogs with surgically-made fistulae of the bile duct and the pancreatic duct. The fistulae were cannulated with glass cannulae and pressure was measured by means of a U-pressure gauge. The pressure in the pancreatic duct system of the fasting dog amounted to 10.0–17.8 cm of water. In the common bile duct, pressures of 9.0–15.0 cm of water were observed.

In 1953 Wulsin and Siler mobilized the pancreatic main duct, detached it from the duodenum, and sutured it up to the abdominal wall. Thus, follow-up studies on intraductal pancreatic pressure could be made. The daily peak levels varied markedly. The average pressure level amounted to 40.0 cm of water, and in one animal a peak level of 82.5 cm of water was observed.

In 1958 Menguy et al., studied the intraductal pressure of the pancreatic duct and the bile duct in 27 dogs. They found an average pancreatic duct pressure of about 14.0 cm of water. In the bile duct the pressure varied from 0–15.8 cm. Dogs that had previously been subjected to cholecystectomy presented an obviously increased bile duct pressure.

According to Davenport's studies (1971), the pancreatic duct pressure in fasting dogs amounts to 2.3–16.7 cm of water. In all dogs the bile duct pressure was found to be lower than the pancreatic duct pressure.

These complicated studies, while necessitating surgery, could not be applied to man for a routine examination. Hess (1969) developed a peroperative routine examination. A cannula is introduced peroperatively into the common bile duct, allowing the surgeon to determine the pressure level, which is required to overcome the resistence of the papilla. The examination is performed peroperatively under fluoroscopic control. The normal biliary duct pressure amounted to 10–15 cm of water. In stenosis of the common bile duct or of the papilla, high pressure levels were observed. Pressures exceeding 40 cm of water indicate occlusion.

Ryan et al. (1949) studied bile duct pressure in a man presenting a traumatic outer biliary fistula. The patient showed pressure levels of about 15 cm of water. White et al. (1964) recorded the pancreatic duct pressure in an 80-year-old female patient who had the pancreatic tail resected for removal of a tumor. A polyethylene cannula was left in the transsected pancreatic duct and the duct pressure was recorded continuously for 10 days. The pressure averaged between 7–12 cm of water. Those authors were the first to observe the effect of respiration on the tracings.

A new road was found by Vondrasek and Eberhart in 1974. These authors tried to record the intraductal pressure endoscopically by the open-tip method. They used a catheter with a sideward sensor attached to the catheter wall 1 mm away from the tip. The sensor consisted of two silicone elements in a semibridge circuit, which were attached to a diaphragm.

These authors found that after application of glucagon, the intraductal pressure ranged between 29.38 and 97.89 mm of water. After stimulation with pancreozymin it increased to 45.95–140.12 mm. The shortcoming of this technique seems to be the lack of position control of the tip of the cannula. The examiner cannot be absolutely sure that the cannula is in an intrapapillary or an intraductal position.

With regard to the above-mentioned difficulties, the authors have developed a simple technique for measuring the intraductal pressure of the pancreatic and the common bile ducts, which allow them to get reproducible results under standardized conditions.

5.7.1 Method

The examinations were performed with the patient on his left side under exactly the same conditions and the same medication as in ERPC. Metal-tipped Teflon cannulae with an inner diameter of 1.0 mm and an outer diameter of 1.6 mm were used. After cannulation of the papilla for exact localization, selective pressure measurement was performed.

As a measuring instrument, the authors used the Hellige imput amplifier LA 20603499 combined with the Statham pressure sensor P 32BB. The pressure was continuously recorded by the Hellige compensatory curve-drawing recorder B 140 (Pen Recorder).

The pressure sensor, a mechanical-electric converter that is connected to the cannula, can be considered the main device. The pressure acts upon a diaphragm. Pressure changes lead to diaphragm oscillations that are converted into proportional electric signals by means of a bridge circuit. The initial level of the amplified signals amounts to 1 V. Prior to each examination, the pressure is adjusted too corresponding to atmospheric pressure.

The pressure values are indicated both by an indicating instrument, in centimeters of water, and by a compensatory curve-drawing recorder. Zero position as well as the deflection of the indicator needle are individually adjustable. The 30 cm H_2O scale of the Imput amplifier was sufficient in almost all cases. Only occasionally was the 60-cm H_2O scale needed. In all measurements the integrated mean pressure values were recorded. Thus, unwanted effects such as artificial waves were eliminated without suppressing relevant pressure changes, such as changes due to respiration movement.

For exact pressure measurements, the tip of the cannula must be at the same level as the pressure sensor. However, since the distance between the tip of the cannula and the x-ray table cannot be exactly assessed, the sensor was adjusted to a reproducible referring point in each patient. According to the site of the pancreas, the processus spinosus of the first lumbar vertebra was chosen as a referring point.

5.7.2 Measuring Errors

Measuring errors, which may be due to the technique or not least to the varying secretory activity of the individual's pancreas, must be taken into consideration.

1. As the catheter does not completely tighten the papilla, a certain amount of juice runs off between the catheter and the sphincter into the duodenum during the examination.

2. In the case of increased secretion, the amount of juice cannot be determined.

3. The catheter itself constitutes a certain barrier to the flow of juice. However, the authors did not observe a considerable influence on the intraductal pressure. This could be proved by control studies with opened and closed connectors.

4. Further inaccuracy is given by the fact that the sensor can only be approximately adjusted to the level of the pancreas.

5. It could be shown that the measured pressure values changed when the opening of the catheter was occluded by the duct wall. Yet, such a condition can easily be recognized by the characteristic continuous decrease of pressure.

5.7.3 Characteristic Pressure Tracings

Apart from the fact that the average pressure is higher in the pancreatic duct than in the common bile duct, the pattern of the pressure tracing of the two duct systems do not substantially differ from one another. Thus, in the isolated case, the tracings do not indicate whether the intrapancreatic or intrabiliary pressure is recorded. Reliable differentiation can only be made by injection of contrast material and fluoroscopic position control or by radiograms. Thus, the description of a characteristic pressure tracing applies to both duct systems.

There are two basic patterns of pressure tracings. Both of them show respiratory movements of only a few millimeters of water. The difference between expiration and inspiration normally averages between 0.2–0.6 cm of water. During maximal inspiration the pressure is raised to 8.0 cm. However, as soon as respiration normalized, the pressure immediately dropped back to normal. Apart from these respiratory movements, the following two basic patterns can be differentiated:

1. The pattern of slight undulations: These tracings show slight, slow pressure changes with a constant average pressure (Fig. 34). The waves are flat and show a maximal range of 2 cm of water. The changes from minimum to maximum values are slow.

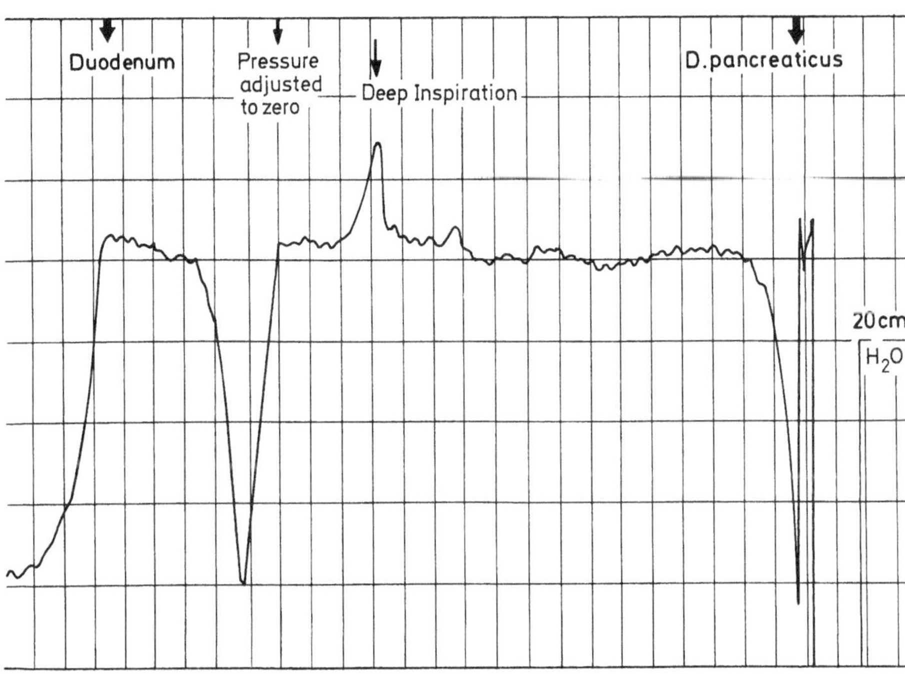

Fig. 34. Characteristic pressure tracing with fine waves measured in pancreatic duct. Low amplitudes with maximum of 2 cm of water. Characteristic increase in pressure during deep inspiration

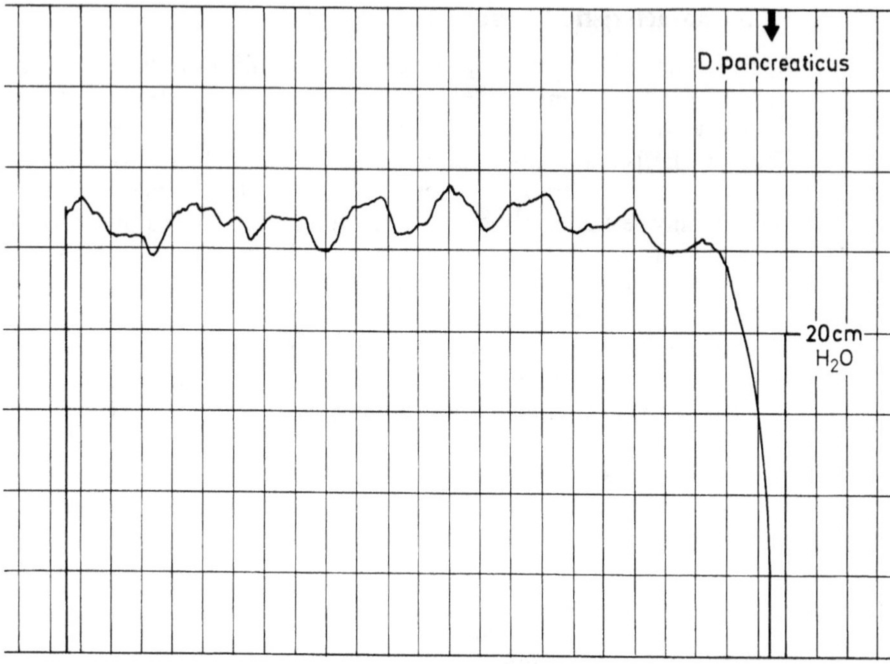

Fig. 35. Characteristic pressure tracing with coarse undulations measured in pancreatic duct. Amplitude can amount to 4 cm of water

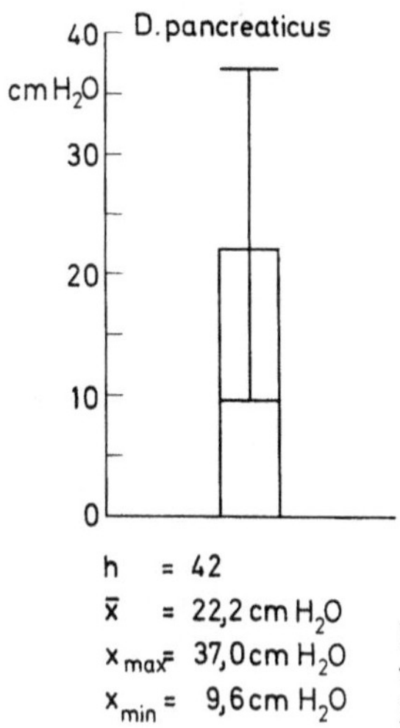

Fig. 36. Diagrams of mean pressure in pancreatic duct with standard deviation. Mean pressure amounts to 22.2 cm of water

2. The pattern of coarse undulations: These tracings show a quick increase and drop in pressure. The difference between maximum and minimum values may amount to several centimeters of water (Fig. 35). A sudden drop in pressure may be due to:

1. Slipping back of the catheter into the duodenum. This can be corrected endoscopically.

2. Incorrect position of the catheter tip. It may be positioned too close to the duct wall, which occludes its opening. The correct pressure is found by correcting the position of the catheter.

5.7.4 Pressure Values in the Pancreatic Duct

In the normal pancreatic duct system the authors found an average pressure of 22.2 cm of water with a standard deviation of ±7.3 cm of water (Fig. 36). A maximum pressure of 37.0 cm of water was found; the minimum pressure was 9.6 cm. In pathologic conditions one can find normal increased or reduced pressure values, depending on the kind and the stage of the lesion. Yet, transitional values are possible. The cases of advanced chronic pancreatitis and chronic relapsing pancreatitis show obviously reduced pressure values, which can drop to zero cm of water in advanced conditions.

In stenosis or occlusions due to carcinoma, the pressure values are markedly reduced in the segment downstream from the lesion and with transient values.

As a rule, papillary stenosis leads to increased pressure values depending on the stage of the lesion.

5.7.5 Pressure Values in the Common Bile Duct

In the common bile duct the pressure averages 12.0 cm of water (Fig. 37). The maximum pressure amounted to 17.0 cm of water, the minimum pressure was 7.3 cm. Hence, a standard deviation of ±3.5 cm. Patients with radiologically proven calculi in the gallbladder did not show a relevant deviation of the mean pressure values from the pressure in normal duct systems. However, in prepapillary concrements with consecutive, marked retention of bile, the pressure is obviously increased. Thus, other stenosing and infiltrating lesions such as carcinomas

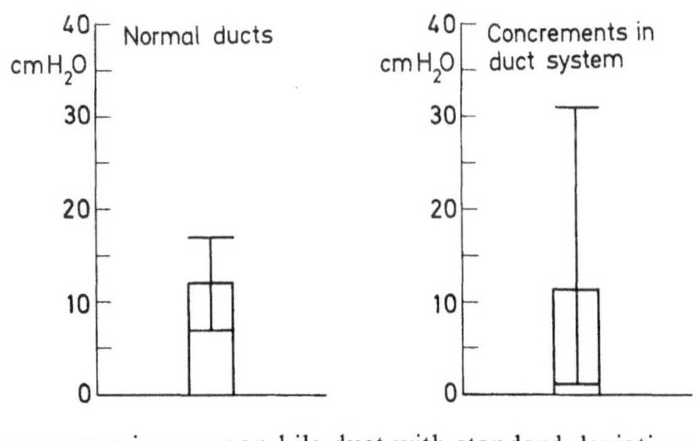

Fig. 37. Diagram of mean pressure in common bile duct with standard deviation. Mean pressure amounts to 12.0 cm of water

of the pancreatic head or tubular stenoses, can lead to a increased pressure in the proximal duct segment. Pressure values of more than 32 cm of water could be found.

5.7.6 Pressure Values in the Duodenum

Intraduodenal pressure measurements were routinely performed at the level of the papilla (Fig. 38). Thus, the function of the device, as well as the position of the catheter tip, could be checked. The intraduodenal pressure mainly depends on the duodenal peristalsis; consequently it is quite variable. It averages 5.3 cm of water with a maximum of 10.9 cm and a minimum of 0.6 cm. The standard deviation is ±2.7 cm. According to the authors' experience, it seems to be useful to perform pressure measurements of both duct systems in combination with ERPC. The pressure measurement studies in the authors' case material as well as in an identical group of patients showed that in the pancreatic duct system the mean pressure is obviously higher than in the common bile duct or in the duodenum. The different pressure levels in the two duct systems, which are well known from animal experiments reported on in the literature, may prevent a reflux under normal conditions. However, the above-mentioned studies resulted in rather different findings as to the height of the intraductal pressure values. Harms (1927) has already demonstrated that those results cannot be compared since the pancreas of the dog has several ducts opening into the duodenum. The mean basic pressure of 22.2 cm of water that has been found by the authors is generally much lower than the pressure values in dogs. Menguy et al. (1958) report on pressure values that correspond partially to the authors' findings. However, the mean pressure value of 14.0 cm of water is obviously lower than the pressure found in

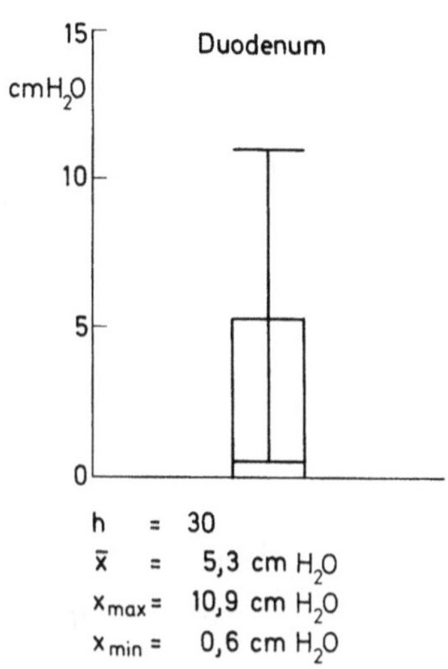

Fig. 38. Diagram of mean pressure at level of papilla. Mean pressure amounts to 5.3 cm of water. There is, however, a distinct variability depending on tonus of duodenal wall

men. On the other hand Wulsin and Siler report a considerably higher mean pressure in dogs amounting to 45.0 cm of water.

In the female patient with resection of the tail of the pancreas, which had been reported on by White et al. (1964), preprandial pressure values of 7–12 cm of water were observed. These pressures are lower than the mean values that had been found by the authors. However, it should be considered that apart from the loss of parenchyma and subsequent diminution of secretion, there was a loss of juice and pressure through the fistula and the papilla. The studies of Vondrasek and Eberhart (1974), which can be best compared to the authors' examinations, revealed pancreatic duct pressure values ranging from 2.9 cm of water to 9.7 cm. They are obviously lower than the pressures that had been observed by the authors. This may be due to the fact—as Vondrasek and Eberhart had already pointed out—that the sideward sensor might have touched the duct wall too closely.

As a rule, the endoscopically studied intraductal biliary pressure in humans is largely identical with the pressure values found in animal experiments. There is obviously a wide range of normal pressure values considering the capability of contraction of the common bile duct. This applies to the mean values of the whole case material as well as to the single case.

In all cases, the pancreatic intraductal pressure was obviously higher than the biliary pressure. The authors also found that the average intraduodenal pressure was obviously lower than the biliary pressure. There is a normal decrease in pressure from the pancreas to the common bile duct and the duodenum, thus preventing reflux under normal conditions. Pathologic changes of the pancreas and the biliary duct may disturb this pressure structure, giving rise to sudden danger. Perhaps pressure measurements may lead to early detection of those risks.

6. The ERPC Roentgenographic Pattern in Changes Due to Age

According to the studies of Milbourn (1959) and Kreel (1973) as well as the authors' studies on 100 retrograde pancreaticograms, the width of the main pancreatic duct increases with age (Fig. 39). Up to the age of 40, the width does not remarkably change. However, beyond the forties the duct may widen and the dilatation may reach 2 mm. Kreel (1975) has found an increasing rate of the ducts caliber of 0.8% per year. According to this author, in advanced age the width of the pancreatic main duct can reach 10 mm in the head of the gland. On the other hand, with increasing age multiple stratification and proliferation of the epithelium may lead to stenosis and even to occlusion of the smaller and larger pancreatic ducts (Becker 1973). Such growth can lead even to the formation of adenomas. The changes of contours and course that the pancreatic main duct undergoes with increasing age are of greater importance for differential diagnosis. Especially in the area of body and tail, the contours and the course of the ducts come to be irregular without pathological findings of the pancreas (Fig. 40). Yet, these changes can be observed in chronic pancreatitis of first and second degree. This implies, that in the individual case,

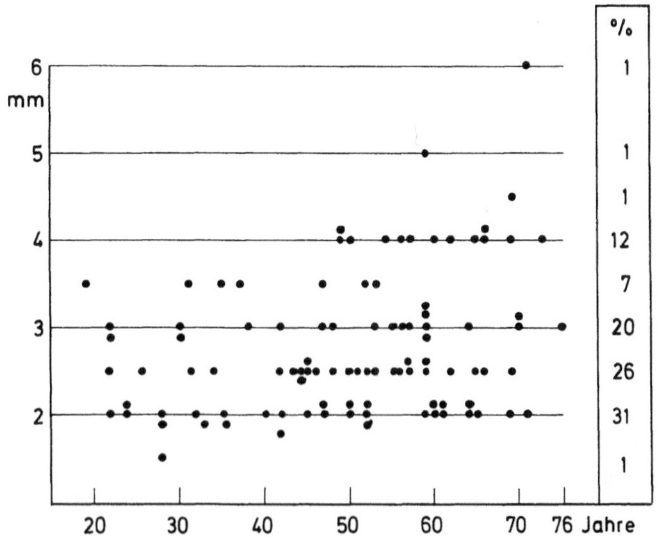

Fig. 39. Width of Wirsung's duct in different age groups

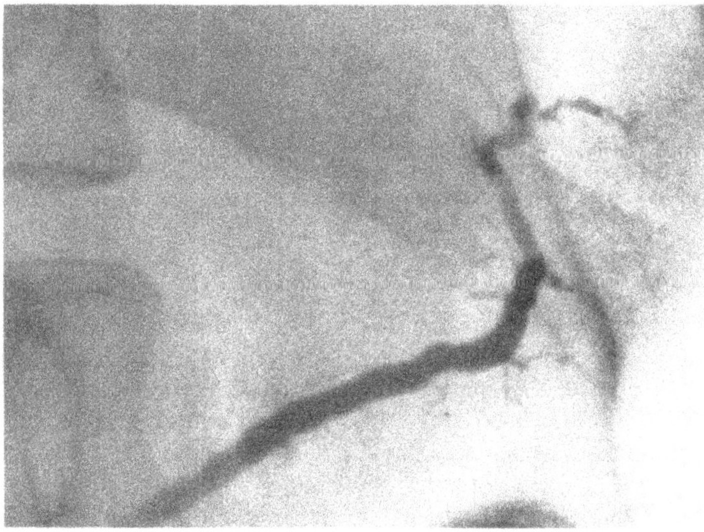

Fig. 40. Changes due to age of Wirsung's duct presenting marginal irregularities in tail of pancreas. Healthy female patient of 54 years

considerable diagnostic problems may arise when these changes are found in an elderly patient, unless no further changes of the duct system or laboratory findings lead to the diagnosis of chronic pancreatitis.

7. The ERPC in Lesions of the Pancreas and the Papilla Duodeni

7.1 Annular Pancreas

Annular pancreas is a rare anomaly. It occurs as a result of failure of a complete rotation to the right of the ventral anlage. Normally, in the early embryonic stage, the pancreas arises from two ventral and one dorsal buds (Fig. 41). The two ventral buds arise from a right- and a left-sided diverticulum of the common bile duct immediately before it opens into the duodenum. The larger dorsal pancreatic diverticulum arises from the foregut and elongates cephalad into the retroperitoneal space. Later on, the left ventral anlage atrophies and fuses with the right one.

When the gut rotates to the right, the dorsal anlage shifts to the left. Differential growth of the duodenal wall shifts the fused ventral

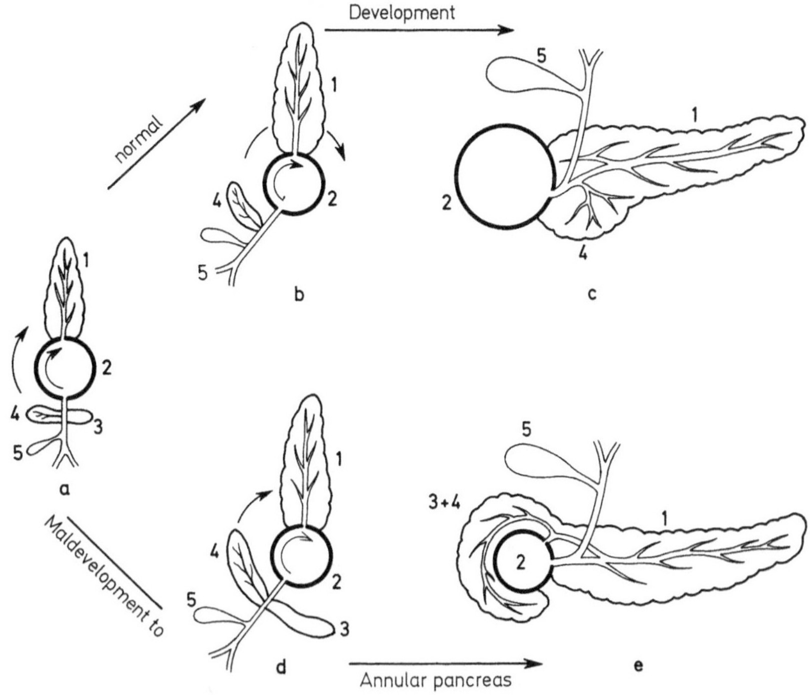

Fig. 41. Normal embryonic development and malformation leading to annular pancreas

anlage to the left, where it fuses with the dorsal one. The ductus pancreaticus major (Wirsung's duct) arises from the ventral anlage, whereas the dorsal anlage often loses its communication with the duodenum and anastomoses with the duct system of the ventral anlage. The main duct of the dorsal anlage is the ductus pancreaticus accessorius (Santorini's duct). If its communication with the duodenum persists, it enters the duodenum at the minor papilla cephalad to the major papilla. At the final stage of embryonic development, the former ventral anlage is situated caudally to the dorsal one and constitutes the uncinate process and the dorsal part of the definite pancreatic head.

There are several theories as to the cause of the annular pancreas. The majority of investigators take the view, that the ring of pancreatic tissue that envelopes the duodenum, comes from the ventral right anlage (Lecco, 1910) or from the left one (Gruber, 1929). The draining duct of this ring may open directly into the duodenum or into the duct of Wirsung (Fehr, 1964).

Annular pancreas gives rise to clinical symptoms mostly in newborns or infants, but only when the pancreatic ring is primarily associated with duodenal stenosis or if the stenosis is secondary to inflammatory swelling of the pancreatic ring. As it is congenital malformation, mostly infants are concerned. Only in slight stenosis can the child reach the age of an adult. The roentgenologic diagnosis can generally be made by demonstration of the duodenum in barium studies. The definite diagnosis is made by ERPC with demonstration of an annular duct system that encircles the duodenum (Bauerle et al., 1972) (Fig. 42a–d).

7.2 Chronic Pancreatitis, Chronic Relapsing Pancreatitis, Calculous Pancreatitis

Since the changes of the duct system secondary to chronic pancreatitis, chronic relapsing pancreatitis, and calculous pancreatitis are almost identical, they will be treated together in this chapter.

Long-persisting inflammation as well as retention of pancreatic juice result in fibrosis and shrinking of the pancreatic parenchyma (Becker, 1973; Nette, 1974). Alterations of the ducts do not develop until the fibrosing and shrinking process encroaches upon the excretory duct system. Hence, it follows that when changes of the duct system can be demonstrated, the inflammatory and scarring process must already have been active for a long time. Consequently, a normal duct system in the initial state of pancreatitis is not a rare finding (Mercadier and Hepp, 1956; Anacker, 1962; Classen et al., 1972; Oi, 1972; and Weiss et al., 1973).

Three different stages can be classified ranging from normal findings to the characteristic aspect of chronic pancreatitis with marked changes of the duct system.

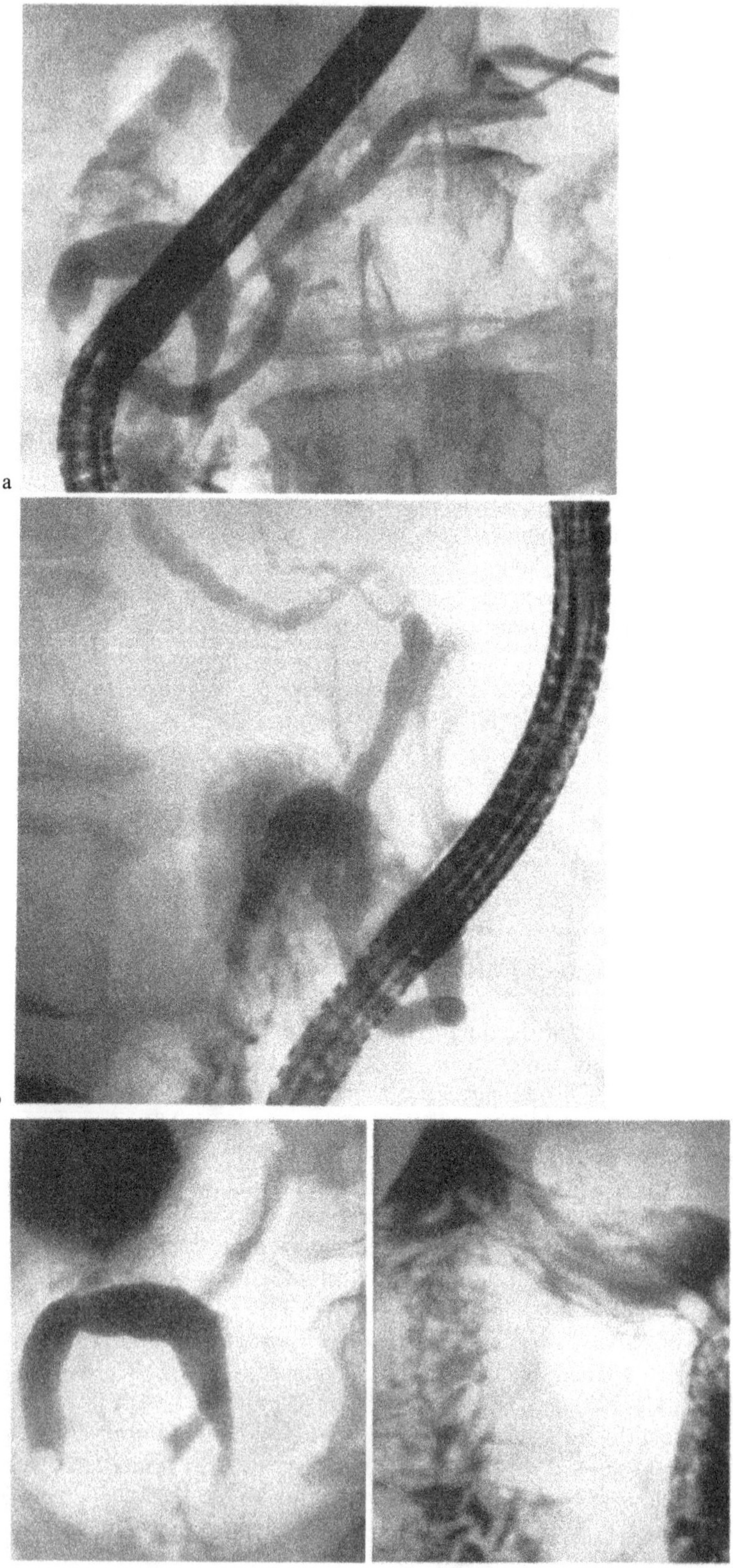

a

b

c

d

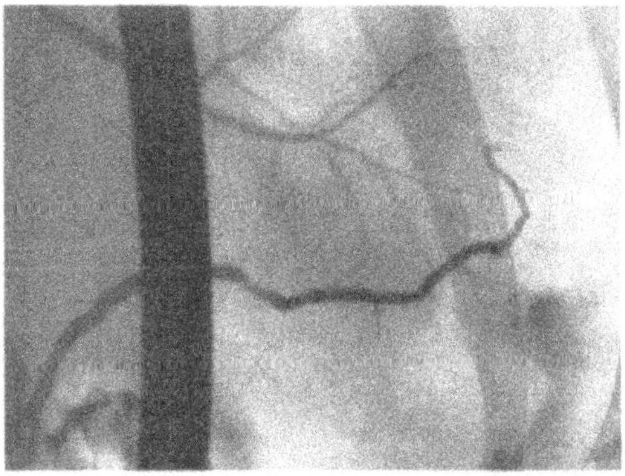

Fig. 43. Irregular course and variations in caliber of Wirsung's duct in pancreatic tail. Side branches are only partially deformed. Accessory finding: overlapping of intrahepatic bile duct in left latero-caudal segment. Left lobe of liver is markedly enlarged, whereas right lobe shows atrophy. Attack of acute pancreatitis 3 years ago. On admission patient presents clinical picture of chronic relapsing pancreatitis with elevation of amylase and lipase activity

1. Stage one: The main duct of the pancreas shows slight marginal irregularities (Fig. 43). Since the shrinking process of the pancreatic parenchyma initially involves the smaller ducts, deformities can be demonstrated at the side branches of Wirsung's duct.

2. Stage two: With long-persisting, progressive changes, the main duct shows irregularities and slight variations in caliber. In this stage, the side branches may already be heavily involved (Fig. 44).

3. Stage three: The distinct aspect of chronic pancreatitis is characterized by severe changes of the entire duct system. In this stage the predominant sign is ectasia of the main duct (Fig. 45) found in more than the half of all cases. On the other hand, the duct may be narrowed in one (Fig. 46) or several (Fig. 47) segments. Solitary or multiple "beading" stenoses may develop (Fig. 48). In *solitary stenosis,* when there are no further changes, difficulties may arise in differentiation from solitary carcinoma or harmless anatomic variants (Fig. 46). For this reason a solitary stenosis should be interpreted as secondary to a chronic pancreatitis only if there are other characteristic inflammatory changes (Weiss et al., 1973).

In this stage the side branches are particularly tortuous and clubby (Fig. 48a), sometimes combined with cystic dilatations. The emptying time of contrast medium is prolonged (Fig. 48b). This may be due in part to the greater quantity of dye needed for filling. Moreover,

◄ Fig. 42a–d. Retrograde pancreaticogram in annular pancreas. Annular course of Wirsung's duct in a.p. view (a) and in lateral view (b). Endoscope marks course of descending duodenum. After removal of instrument, oblique view shows annular segment which encircles descending duodenum (c). Upper gastrointestinal barium study reveals no stenosis (d)

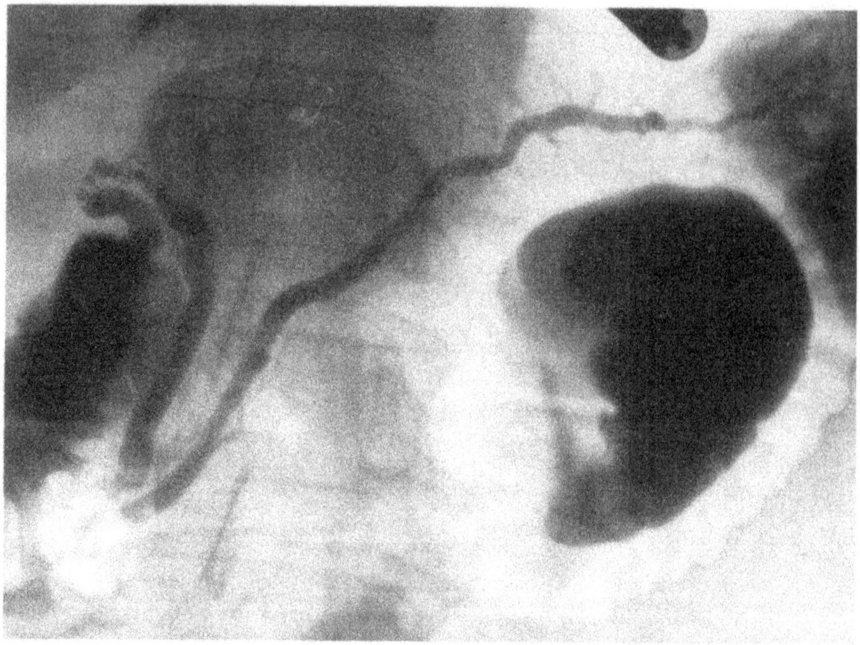

Fig. 44. Somewhat irregular course of Wirsung's duct which shows slight variations in caliber and tail of gland. Moderate ectasia of side branches in case of chronic pancreatitis of low degree

the contrast medium may remain for some time in the dilated segments of the involved ducts. Okuda et al. (1973) observed in 10 cases of chronic pancreatitis *delayed emptying,* the average time being 26.5 min – an extremely long period.

In a persisting chronic inflammatory process the pancreatic parenchyma shrinks whereas the main duct widens simultaneously. According to Nette (1973) these two factors, shrinking and widening, permit the degree of the disease to be assessed. The author has developed a ratio between the size of the gland in square centimeters and the width of the main duct. This gland size duct width ratio, normally 1:20, decreases in inverse proportion to the degree of pancreatitis. Since in a high percentage of cases the *common bile duct* runs inside the head of the gland, it *is involved* by the shrinking process of the parenchyma secondary to chronic pancreatitis. Generally stenoses develop; their contours are smooth and mostly concentric in contrast to those secondary to carcinoma of the pancreatic head. Classen and Demling (1973) observed such benign stenoses in 16% of 64 cases of chronic pancreatitis (Fig. 48c). The authors found only one case of stenosis of the common bile duct with marginal irregularities. However, in this case differential diagnosis did not present difficulties, since the

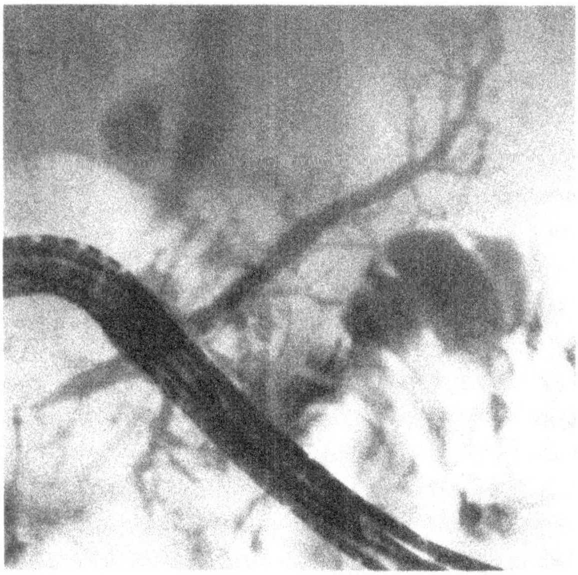

Fig. 45. Chronic pancreatitis with considerable dilatation of Wirsung's duct, rami, and ductuli. Patient suffering from chronic pancreatitis for 8 years

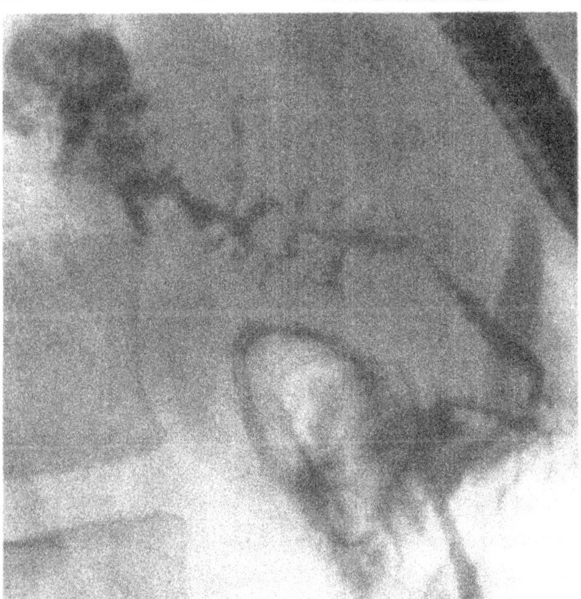

Fig. 46

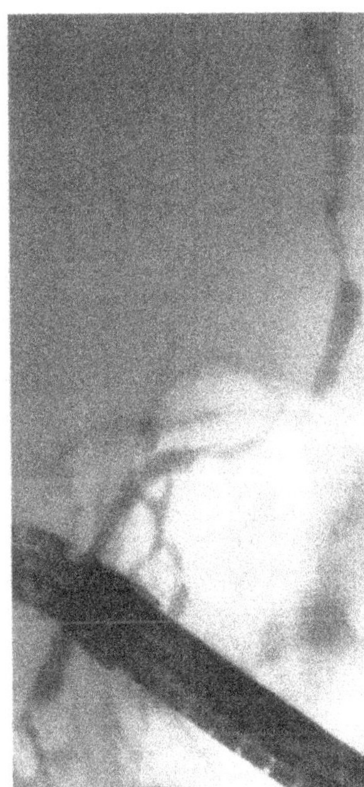

Fig. 47

Fig. 46. Stenosis of Wirsung's duct in body of pancreas. Prestenotic dilatation of all ducts in pancreatic tail. Alcoholic, 24-years-old, whose history began with attack of acute pancreatitis 6 years ago. In following years he suffered from alternating abdominal pain. On admission he presented acute pancreatic attack with elevation of serum lipase to 13,000 mμ/ml, amylase level was 400 mμ/ml

Fig. 47. Several partially long stenoses of Wirsung's duct in case of chronic pancreatitis. Marked deformations of ramus capitis inferior, which is found downstream from stenoses, may serve as criterion for differential diagnosis. Alcoholic, 41-year-old, with chronic pancreatitis

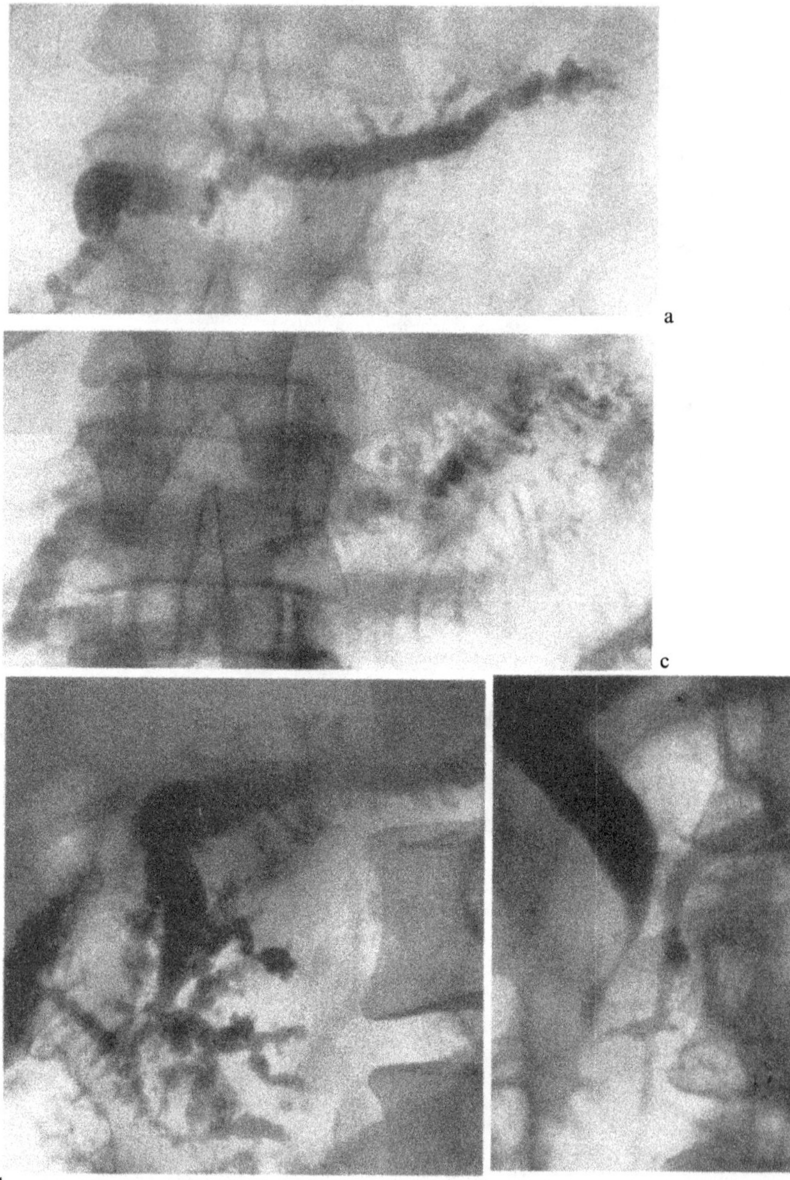

Fig. 48a–c. Beading of Wirsung's duct. Chronic pancreatitis, ectasia, and annular stenosis of pancreatic main duct. Deformations of side branches. Surgery revealed overall indurated, ragged gland. (a) Patient with chronic pancreatitis for 8 years with marked ectasia presenting to some extent cystic aspect. Deformation of rami and ductuli pancreatici. At surgery pancreas was indurated and ragged. After incision of dilated main duct, numerous calculi were found. A postoperative review of roentgenograms reveals filling defects in some side branches, which might correspond to concrements. (b) Delayed emptying of extremely dilated duct system. Same case as in Fig. a. One hour after injection duct system was still opacified. (c) Stenoses of intrapancreatic segment of common bile duct with smooth borders in chronic pancreatitis. At surgery head of gland was enlarged, entire pancreas was indurated and ragged

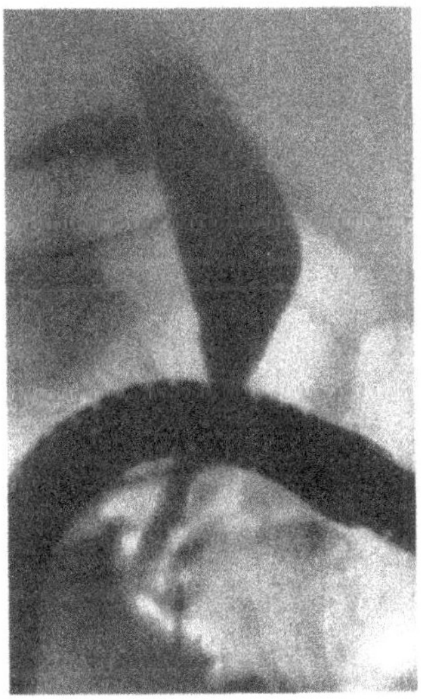

Fig. 49

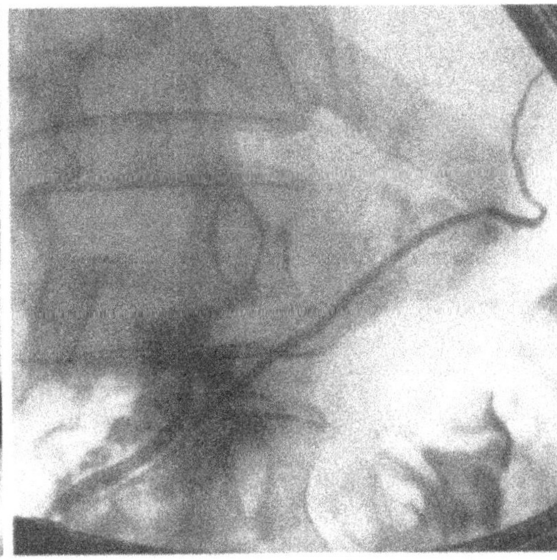

Fig. 50

Fig. 49. Slightly irregular stenoses of common bile duct with marked prestenotic dilatation in chronic pancreatitis. In this case differential diagnosis did not present difficulties since pancreatic duct system showed changes which were obviously due to inflammatory origin (cf. Fig. 48)

Fig. 50. "Premature" acinar filling. Opacification is distinct above all in pancreatic head. Otherwise normal duct system in chronic pancreatitis

changes of the pancreatic duct system were obviously suggestive of chronic pancreatitis (Fig. 49).

Since the advent of peroperative pancreaticography, the picture of premature patchy filling of the parenchyma with dye has become well-known (Doubilet et al., 1955, Léger, 1961, Mercadier and Hepp, 1956). This phenomenon, described as "image maculaire en nappe," was interpreted as a symptom of a localized pancreatitis. A striking feature of this phenomenon is the fact that, apart from slight ectasia of the main duct, the other ducts are obviously normal (Fig. 50). Thus, induced by normal injection pressure, this premature parenchymal opacification is in the main the only sign indicative of pancreatitis. The phenomenon disappears when the acute inflammatory process subsides.

The premature diffusion of dye into the acini may be explained by loss of semipermeability of the ductal epithelium in the affected area, where the pancreatic juice contains trypsin instead of trypsinogen (Doubilet et al.). Diffusion of contrast material, however, can also be provoked in the normal pancreas by increased injection pressure. This can occur in retrograde pancreaticography when the tip of the catheter tightens the orifice of the duct. In such a condition, called "overfilling," the patient experiences pain or a sensation of pressure. A premature diffusion of dye should be judged as a pathologic finding provided the patient does not feel pain and the catheter does not tighten the orifice of the duct preventing contrast material from flowing back into the duodenum.

According to the authors' observations, parenchymal opacification did not induce relapse of the inflammatory process, nor were amylase levels elevated.

Table 3. Changes of the pancreatic duct system in chronic pancreatitis or chronic relapsing pancreatitis

	Authors' case material (1974)	Findings reported by Oi (1972a)
Normal findings	4	6
Marginal irregularities	76	7
Deformation of side branches	38	6
Irregular course	20	2
Variations in caliber	37	
Ectasia	52	
Stenosis	24	4
Changes of common bile duct	18	
Premature opacification of parenchyma	8	
Calculi	7	3
$n=$	83	9

In the authors' cases ectasia, marginal irregularities, and deformities of the side branches are the most frequent signs; these findings are in accordance with those reported on in the literature. What has been said about solitary stenoses applies as well to all other signs: a single isolated sign is inconclusive. The more distinct a sign is and the more each sign is combined with another, the more accurate the diagnosis will be.

Table 4. Relation between the stage of chronic pancreatitis and duration of history

History	Stage I	Stage II	Stage III
0–2 years	46	8	0
2–5 years	32	24	19
>5 years	2	41	46

According to Nette's studies (1973) pancreatitis originates in focal areas. In beginning pancreatitis the pancreaticogram reveals slight changes of the ducts that may be spread over the entire duct system or localized to a certain segment. In the authors' case material, mostly localized lesions were found to affect the pancreatic tail.

In the authors' case material the efficiency of ERPC in the diagnosis of chronic pancreatitis is found to be rather high. Of 83 cases of chronic pancreatitis confirmed by laboratory findings, clinical course, or surgery, the correct diagnosis could be established by ERPC in 79 cases (95%). In 4 cases the diagnoses were found to be false. These findings are consistent with those by Romani et al., who reported on 26 cases of chronic pancreatitis. The diagnosis could be established by ERPC in 25 cases; in 1 case the diagnosis was false negative. A comparative study on the efficiency of ERPC, arteriography, echography, and scintigraphy is given in Chapter 9.

Calculous Pancreatitis

In ERPC two kinds of calculous pancreatitis can be observed; with calculi in the duct system and without. These two patterns cannot be differentiated on the abdominal plain film.

a) Calculous pancreatitis with calculi in the duct system.

Calculi in the duct system can be the result of an inflammatory process or the cause of a relapsing inflammation. Generally they are situated in the main duct and can easily be demonstrated as filling defects (Fig. 51). For the most part one can observe dilatation of the

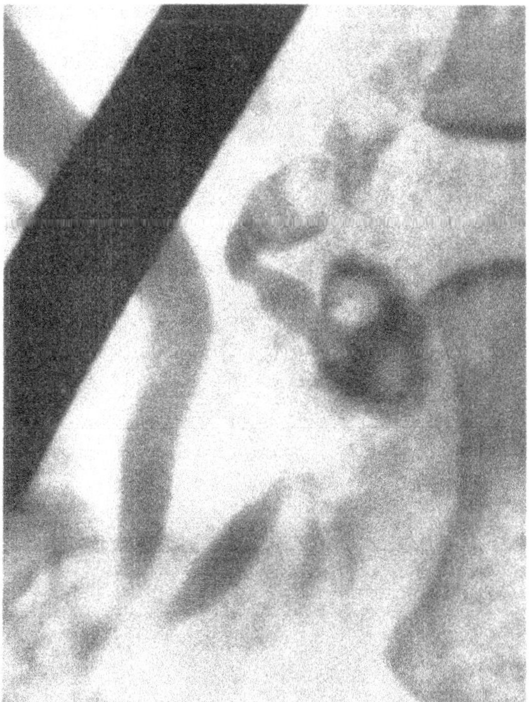

Fig. 51. Multiple calculi in slightly dilated pancreatic duct and in side branches with cystic dilatations. Patient, 37-years-old, with acute relapsing pancreatitis. For 1 year urine diastase level 4 times higher than normal

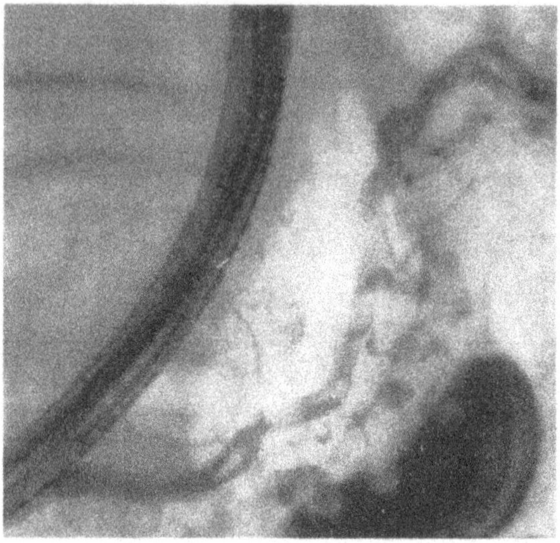

Fig. 52. Multiple oval concrements in dilated Wirsung's duct. They can be demonstrated as contrast filling defects. Distinct ectasia of side branches

main duct, which may be interpreted as the result of a temporary partial obstruction caused by one of the calculi (Fig. 52). If the papilla is obstructed by a concrement, ERPC must fail and pancreaticography must be performed peroperatively.

b) Calculous pancreatitis without calculi in the demonstrable duct system.

Certain cases present obvious pancreatic calcifications on plain films. In ERPC, however, there may be no concrements in the opacified duct system (Fig. 53a, b). Oi (1972a) reported on six cases of pancreaticolithiasis, in three of which calculi could not be demonstrated in the duct system. Since in these cases the ducts present no pathologic changes, the calcifications may be situated in the smallest terminal ends of the canaliculi and ductuli or in the parenchyma, and thus do not manifest themselves on ERPC.

Post-traumatic pancreatitis with occlusion or rupture of the pancreatic duct and consecutive edema of the pancreatic fluid with inflammation (Becker, 1973) can hardly be demonstrated on ERPC.

Stenoses of the pancreatic duct, which are of other origin, can lead to similar sequelae. The authors observed a patient that presented with a stenosis of the main duct due to an aneurism of the superior mesenteric artery. This finding was similar to the observations on post-mortem studies that are reported by Kreel (1975). There were considerable prestenotic deformations of the duct system such as in chronic pancreatitis (Fig. 54). Since the stenosis was combined with displacement, the finding was highly suggestive of carcinoma until surgery revealed the definite cause of the lesion.

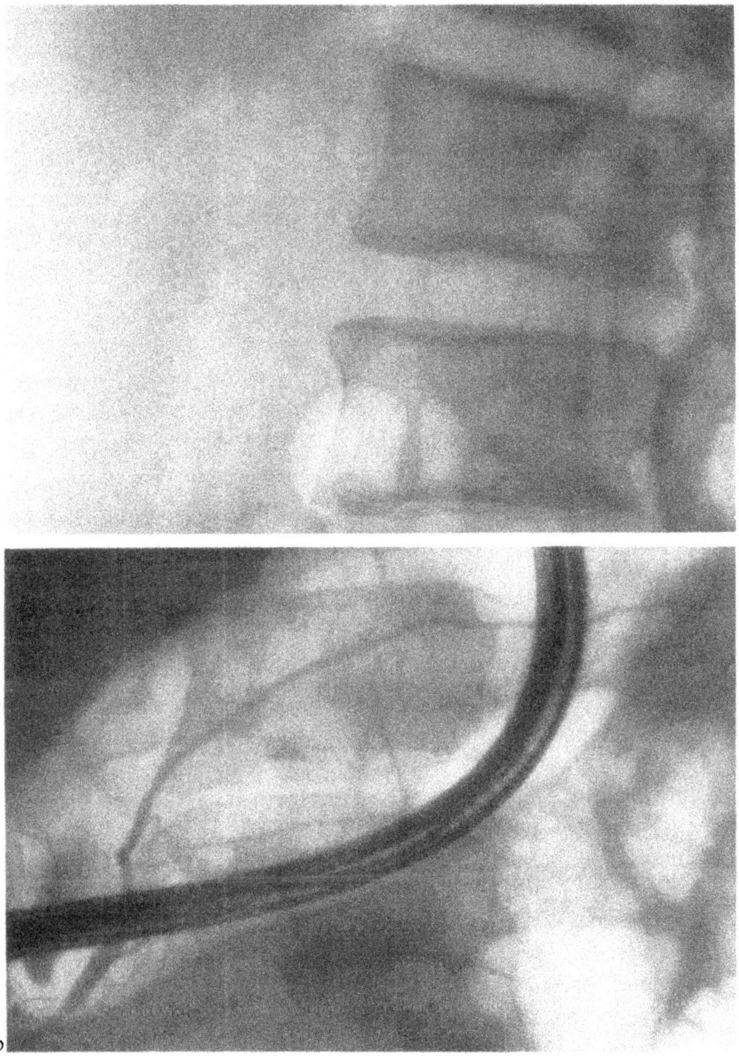

a

b

Fig. 53a and b. Patchy calcific densities in pancreas on abdominal plain film (a). Duct system does not reveal calculi (b)

7.3 Necrotizing Lesions and Pseudocysts

Radiologic visualization of necrotizing cavities and pancreatic pseudocysts has already been performed as peroperative pancreaticography (Patel and Lataste, 1954; Doubilet and Mulholland, 1956; Doubilet et al., 1959; and Anacker, 1962). In these conditions ERPC presents several advantages: A reliable diagnosis of necrotizing lesions or pseudocysts can be established, indication for surgical intervention can be

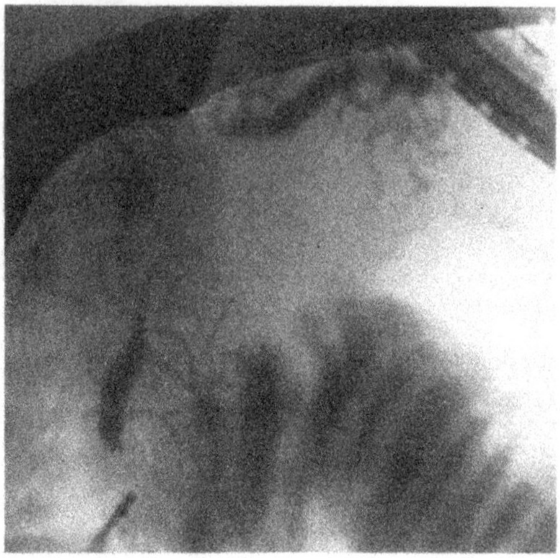

Fig. 54. Stenosis and displacement of pancreatic duct. Prestenotic ectasia of Wirsung's duct and side branches. Pancreatic carcinoma was suspected. Surgery revealed aneurysmatic dilatation of superior mesenteric artery, which led to stenosis

assessed, and planning of surgical intervention can be made prior to operation. Depending on the condition of the duct system in the neighborhood of an abscess or a pseudocyst, one can decide preoperatively on the nature of operation to be performed. A simple cleansing or draining of an abscess, a marsupialization, or an anastomosis between the duct system and the small bowel, can be planned contingent on the draining function of the duct system. However, demonstration of a necrotic cavity is an absolute indication for surgical intervention within 24 h after filling, or with a delay of 2 to 3 days if the cavity is quickly emptied (Seifert et al., 1974).

A pancreatic necrosis occurs in hemorrhagic necrotizing pancreatitis or primarily in the acute condition or in an acute attack of chronic relapsing pancreatitis. Tryptic liquefaction of the parenchyma gives rise to the formation of a cavity with possible sequestration. Tryptic liquefaction leads to rupture of the ducts, allowing pancreatic juice to escape into the cavity or beyond the confines of the gland, forming a pseudocyst. Bleeding into the duct system and through the papilla of Vater into the duodenum is a rare finding. It can be detected by endoscopy.

A necrotizing pancreatic lesion predominates in males in a ratio of about 5 or 6 to 1 (Seifert et al., 1974; Weiss et al., 1975). There is no obvious predominance of localization in the head, body, or tail of the gland.

ERPC reveals the following pathologic changes in necrotizing lesions and pseudocysts.

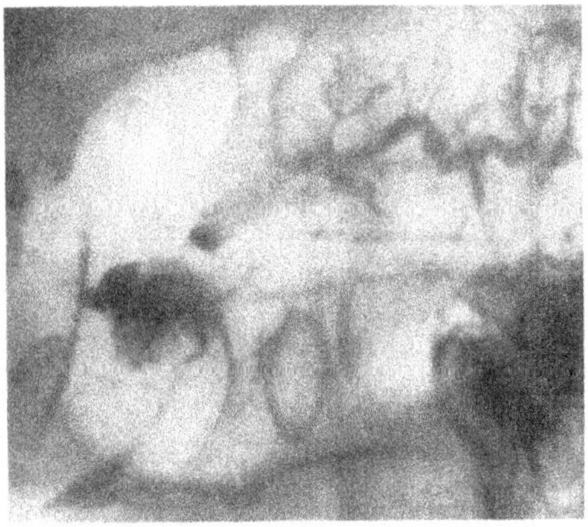

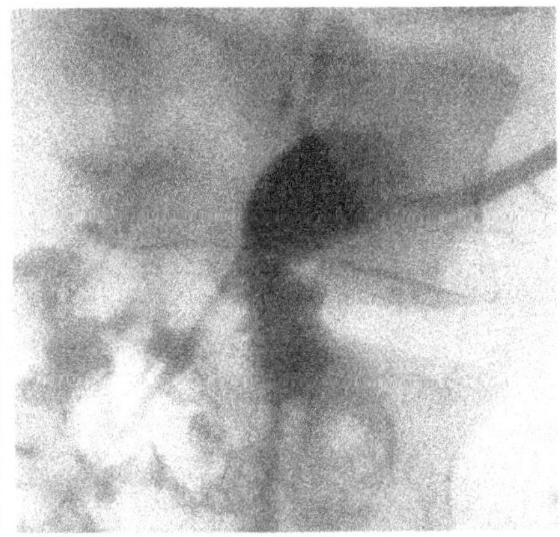

Fig. 55 Fig. 56

Fig. 55. Escape of contrast material into abscess 2.5 cm in size in pancreatic head. Dye seems to escape from stenosed Wirsung's duct. Irregular filling defects in lacunary pooling of dye due to sequestration. Distinct deformation of remnant pancreatic duct system. Stenosis of common bile duct in neighborhood of abscess

Fig. 56. Sideward perforation of pancreatic duct and escape of dye into cavity which extends over nearly whole pancreatic head. Irregular stenosis in vicinity of tryptic perforation

1. Escape of contrast material from the duct system into lacunary cavities
2. Sideward perforation or complete liquefaction of a duct
3. Occlusion of a duct
4. Displacement of a duct
5. Deformation of the remaining duct system
6. Narrowing and displacement of the common bile duct

In addition to these changes one may occasionally find calculi in the pancreatic main duct as well as in the bile duct. Seifert et al. (1974) diagnosed a cyst by demonstrating a nonopacified area in the parenchyma. However, intentional filling of the acini for parenchymal opacification and demonstration of a filling defect may be rather disquieting because of the significant elevation of amylase and lipase levels.

The most obvious and the most important finding in ERPC is escape of the contrast material from the duct system into an abscess or a pseudocyst, which may be localized in the gland or extend into the retroperitoneal or peritoneal space (Fig. 55). This prevalent symptom is found by all authors (Oi, 1970, Cotton et al., 1972, and Manegold et al., 1974). Of 14 cases the authors saw the symptom in 13 patients, Stender et al. (1974) report on 7 patients out of 10 cases, and Rohrmann et al. (1974) in 62% out of 16 cases.

The tryptic lesion leads to a sideward perforation (Fig. 56) or to a complete liquefaction of the duct (Fig. 57). The contrast material

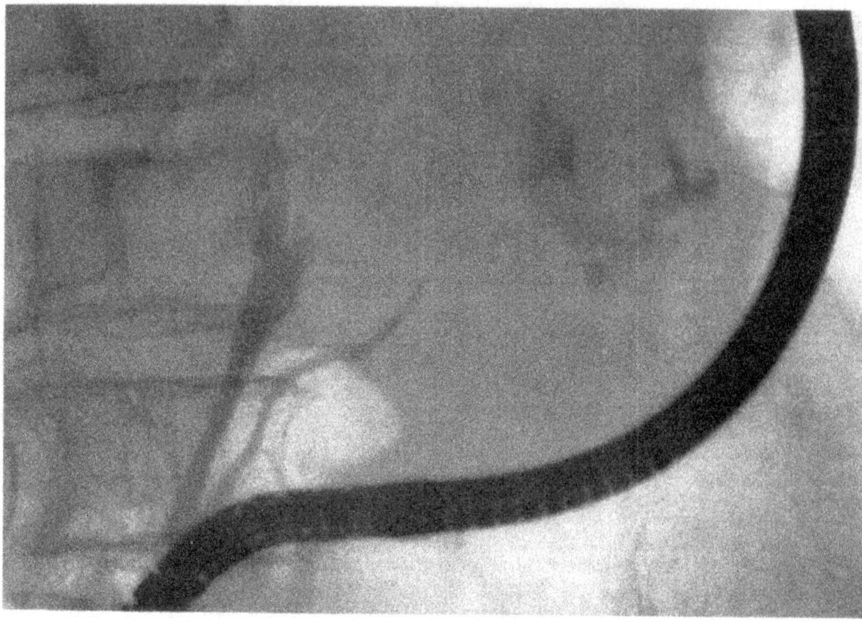

Fig. 57. Complete liquefaction of pancreatic duct in head. Dye escapes into large cavity where it spreads irregularly (pancreatic sequestration) and is quickly diluted. Patient, 71-years-old, with hematemesis. Acute pancreatitis with repeated elevation of amylase activity for 1 week. Tumor in upper abdomen which quickly increases in size to that of child's head

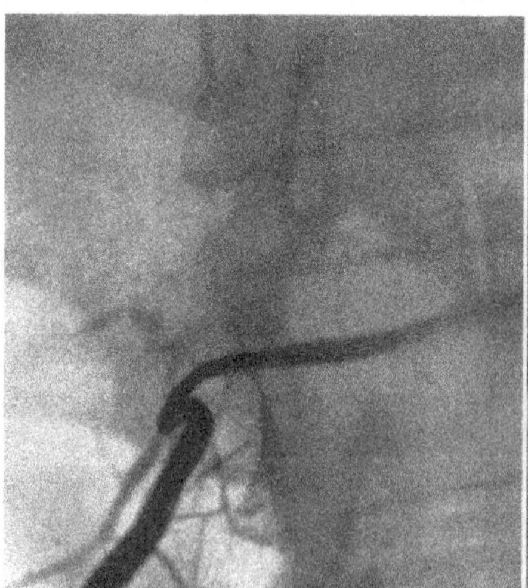

Fig. 58

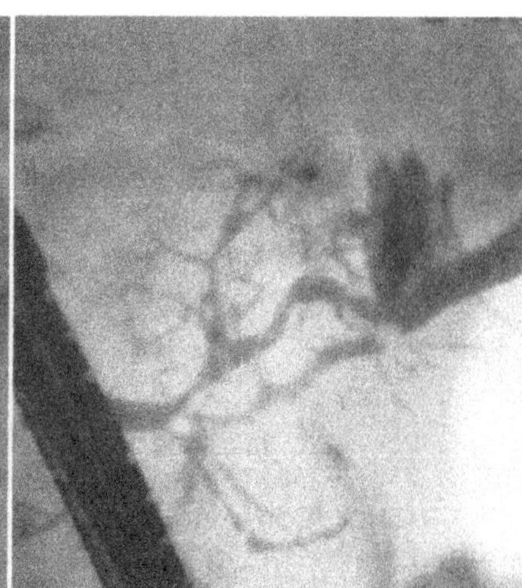

Fig. 59

Fig. 58. Tryptic destruction of numerous small side branches in pancreatic duct

Fig. 59. Tryptic destruction of multiple rami and ductuli in well-localized area of pancreatic body. In neighborhood tryptic necrosis already led to formation of cavity. At surgery abscess was found. Secondary finding: anomalous collateral duct

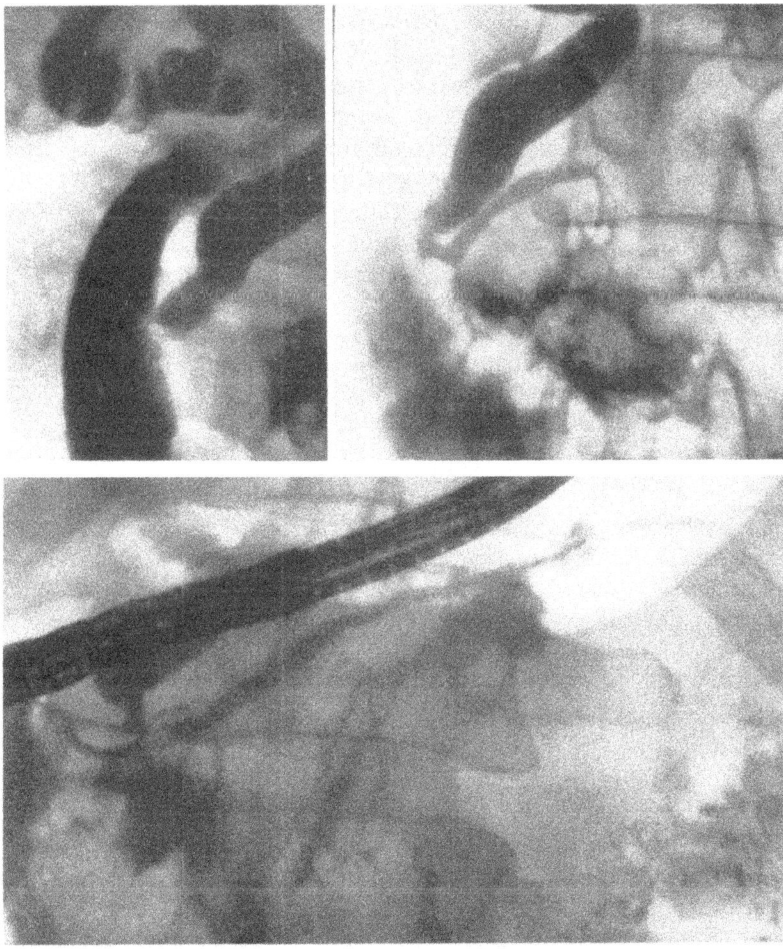

a c

b

Fig. 60a–c. Large postnecrotic cavity fed by perforated ramus capitis inferior (b). Surgery reveals cavity of 5.7 cm situated in pancreatic head and body. It contains a milky liquid and numerous sequestrations. Prepapillary concrement in common bile duct in cholelithiasis (a). In emptying phase only pancreatic duct system was emptied whereas bile ducts remained filled with contrast material. In order to accelerate evacuation, patient was brought to upright position. Due to change of patient's positioning prepapillary concrement passes over into prepapillary segment of pancreatic duct and contrast medium again fills pancreatic duct (bilio-pancreatic reflux), and above all the ramus capitis (b). Repeated escape of dye into cavity. Irregular filling defect in cavity due to pancreatic sequestration (c)

follows the path of the pancreatic juice. In case of a sideward perforation, the whole duct is visualized by the dye that escapes from the sideward leakage into the lesion; in case of complete liquefaction the duct ends in the necrotic cavity. ERPC visualizes the duct ending in the lacunary cavity.

Sometimes one can observe the tryptic lesion in an early stage, when only small ducts in a circumscribed are a are destroyed with a relatively small cavity (Figs. 58 and 59). In such cases the radiologist must give the surgeon an exact localization of the lesion.

The lacunary pooling of contrast material is a common sign indicating pancreatic abscesses, infected necrotic cavities mostly of tryptic origin, as well as pseudocysts secondary to a tryptic pancreatic necrosis resulting in a more or less cleaned and sterile cavity.

The size of the abscesses in the authors' case material ranged from 0.9 to 5.5 cm. The size of the pseudocysts cannot be well assessed because they cannot be exactly delineated. They ranged from 7 to 13.5 cm minimum.

In view of the possible hazards it is not advisable to fill the cavities completely with contrast material. Hence it follows that for differentiation of abscesses from pseudocysts, their different sizes cannot serve as criterian. However, in an abscess cavity one can often visualize irregular filling defects indicating necrotic detritus or sequestration (Fig. 60a, b, c). In pseudocysts the dye is often quickly diluted due to the cyst liquid.

In the healing or scarring process the leakage of the duct may be tightened so that the communication between the duct system and the cavity may be lost. In such conditions ERPC can show complete occlusion of the involved duct. The duct may end in a sharp stop or it may gradually decrease in width (tapered stenosis) (Fig. 61a, b). In such changes, which Cotton and Beales (1974) observed in 4 of 25 cases and Seifert et al. (1974) in 13 of 32 cases, the diagnosis of necrotizing cavity cannot be made by ERPC alone. The pancreatic duct can be displaced and narrowed by abscesses and more distinctly by pseudocysts (Fig. 62a, b). If such a displacement is found combined with deformations of the side branches in the immediate neighborhood of lacunary pooling of dye, the diagnosis can easily be established. However, displacement of a duct without any other pathologic changes is an ambiguous sign. Seifert et al. (1974) observed displacement of ducts in 11 of 32 cases (Fig. 63).

Since necrotizing lesions often develop in the course of acute bouts of relapsing pancreatitis, duct changes secondary to a chronic pancreatitis can often be seen in patients with necrotizing cavities. The authors' case material found four patients who presented changes of the duct system secondary to an advanced stage of chronic pancreatitis; in two cases these deformations were confined to the immediate neighborhood of the abscess.

Coexisting stenoses and displacement of the common bile duct can be interpreted as secondary to a chronic pancreatitis in the same way as inflammatory changes of the pancreatic ducts. They can be found when the pancreatic head or the whole gland are involved.

The more roentgenographic signs can be found, the more precise the differential diagnosis of necrotizing pancreatic lesions will be. A single sign does not present sufficient evidence. Lacunary pooling of contrast material, the most reliable sign, can also be observed in necrotic

Fig. 61 a and b. Perforation of Wirsung's duct and lacunary pooling in pancreatic tail in case of pancreatic necrosis (a). Some months after conservative therapy complete occlusion of Wirsung's duct at segment of previous necrosis (b)

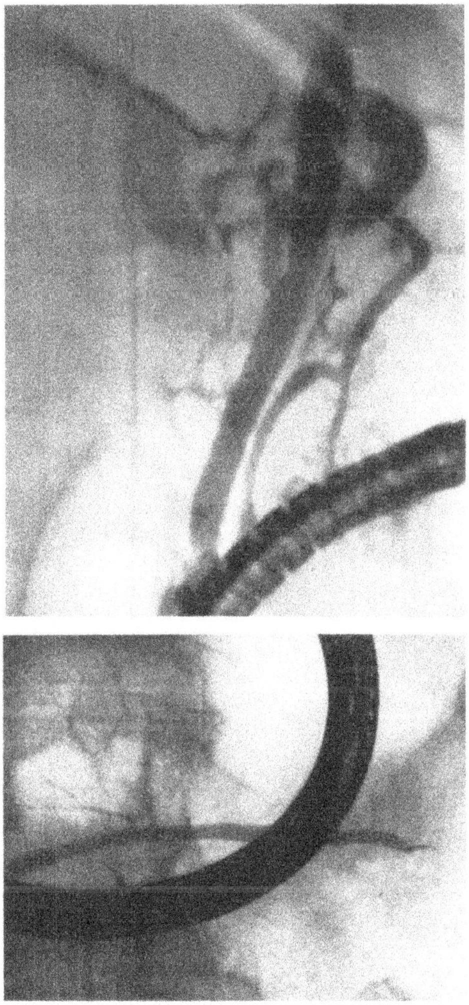

a

b

tumor tissue (Fig. 76a, b). Indeed, deformations similar to those of inflammatory origin can occasionally be observed in carcinoma (Stadelmann et al., 1972). As a rule, however, they are absent. One cannot differentiate pseudocysts from true pancreatic cysts; this is true above all in small cysts with smooth outlines (Seifert et al.). Absence of organ displacement in the vicinity of the cyst and of the neighboring duct segment, presenting no inflammatory changes, is indicative of true cysts (Stender et al., 1974). On the other hand, when a sideward perforation with lacunary pooling of contrast medium is seen in ERPC, one may suspect a pseudocyst.

The most important criterion for differential diagnosis is given by diffusely spread deformations of the duct system, especially of the smaller pancreatic ducts. If a clear diagnosis cannot be made by means

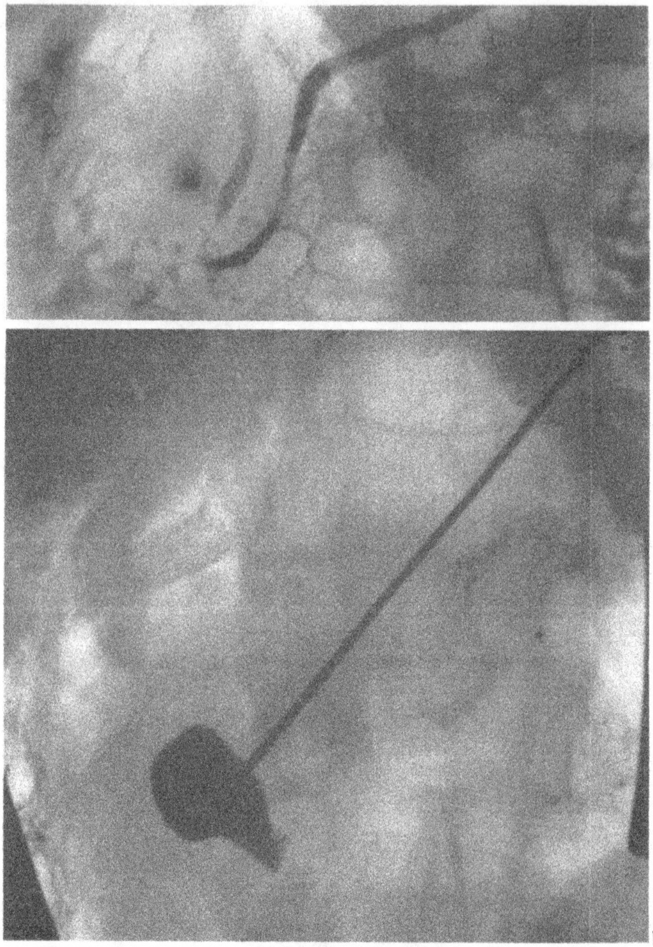

Fig. 62a and b. Small pancreatic abscess with lacunary pooling of dye in head of neighboring segments of pancreatic duct and common bile duct showing slight displacement and stenosis. Slight marginal irregularities of pancreatic duct; borders of bile duct are smooth. Moderate deformations of rami and ductuli pancreatici. Surgery reveals thickening and induration of pancreatic head. According to findings in ERPC, a blind puncture is performed in surgery. Second attempt is successful: a milky fluid is aspirated. Cavity is filled with contrast material for peroperative radiologic control. Then cavity is opened and drained (courtesy Dr. Scholze)

of ERPC, the other clinical and roentgenologic symptoms must give supplementary aid.

7.4 Papillary Stenosis and Papillary Spasm

In papillary stenosis and papillary spasm ERPC enables us to reveal in detail morphologic and functional changes that can only be suspected

Fig. 63. Pancreatic pseudocyst with narrowing and backward displacing of duct of Wirsung ▶

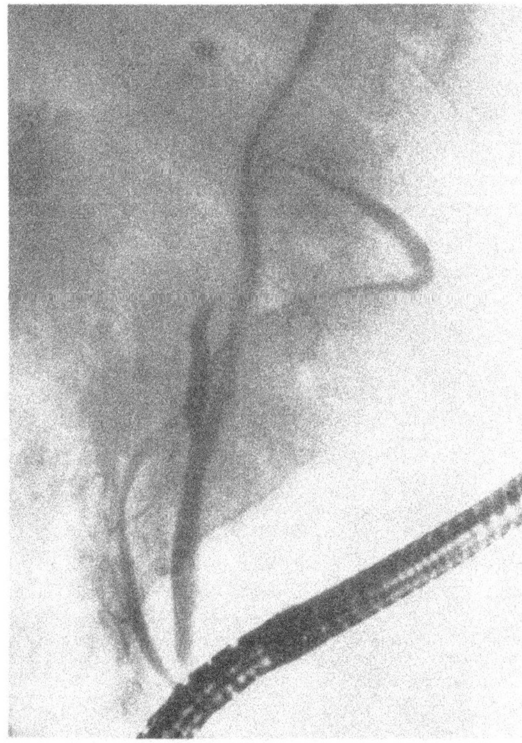

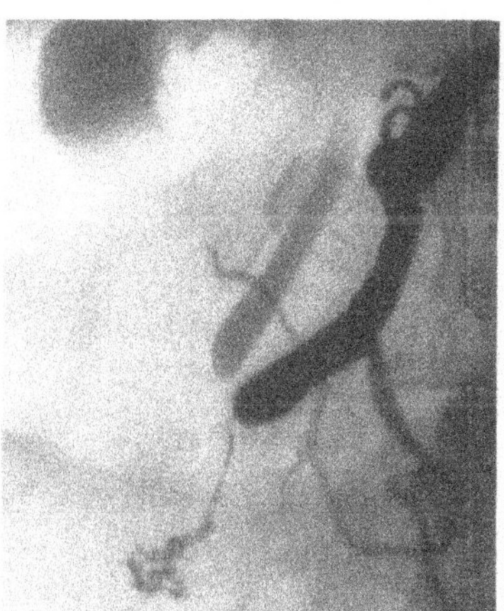

Fig. 64

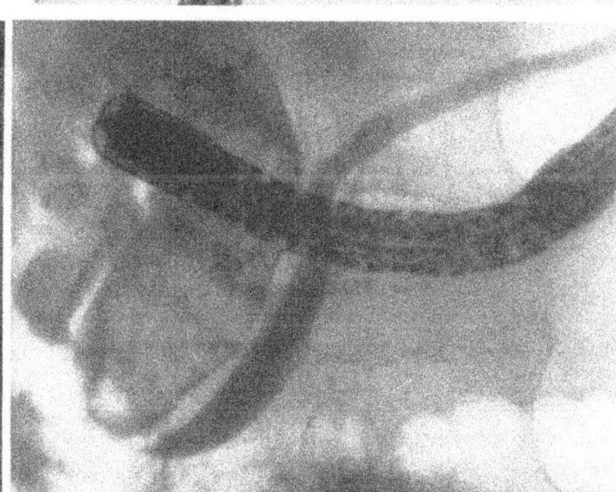

Fig. 65

Fig. 64. Papillary stenosis with narrowing of prepapillary segment of pancreatic duct, which is relatively more dilated than common bile duct. Delayed emptying which lasts for 12 min. [Absence of characteristic phases, continous and delayed draining of dye into duodenum]

Fig. 65. Papillary stenosis with marked ectasia of common bile duct, which contains numerous concrements of different size. Prepapillary segment is not demonstrated but terminal segment of pancreatic duct communicates with common bile duct. Thus biliary-pancreatic or pancreo-biliary reflux is possible

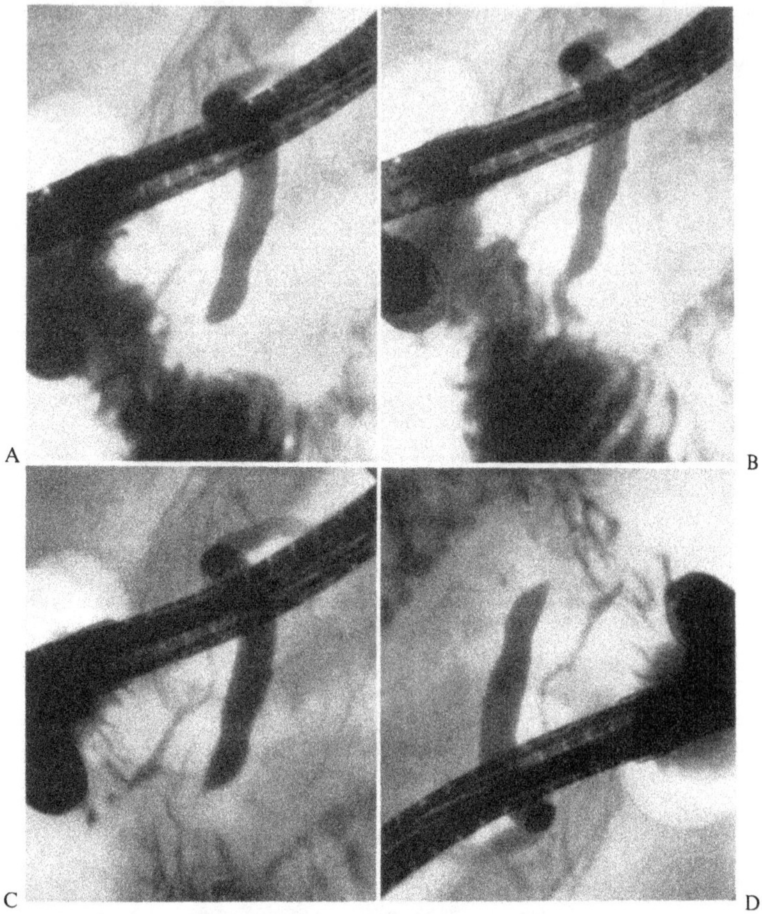

Fig. 66. Papillary stenosis with delayed emptying. Emptying time lasts more than 7 min. Papillary motility could be observed such as emptying phase (*D*), retraction phase (*A*) and recreation phase (*D*). As often as duodenal peristalsis ebbed, pancreatic main duct emptied into duodenum. On the other hand, there was contraction of sphincter muscles during peristaltic contraction of duodenum

in transvenous cholangiography. According to the anatomic conditions, the stenosis may involve in various degrees the common terminal duct segment, the distal end of the common bile duct, or the distal end of the pancreatic duct. This mechanism gives rise to the well-known clinical patterns of biliary tract lesions when the common bile duct is involved, of excretory pancreopathy when the pancreatic duct is involved, and finally of the combination of both conditions if the common segment of the two duct systems is affected. The following morphologic and functional changes can be demonstrated by ERPC:

The common segment of the two duct systems is generally narrowed to a filiform stenosis with smooth or irregular contours; its course can be twisted or straight (Figs. 64, 67a). Proximal to the stenosis

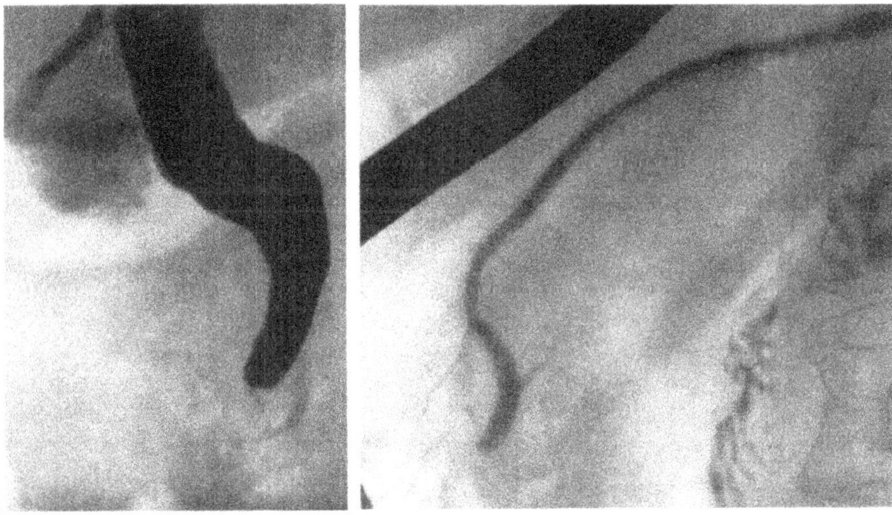

a b

Fig. 67a and b. Papillary stenosis; common bile duct is mainly involved. Cirrhosis of gallbladder, which contains several calculi (a). Delayed emptying, though papillary motility seems to be unchanged. Minor stenosis of intrapapillary segment of pancreatic duct with subsequent minor prestenotic ectasia. Additional draining through Santorini's duct via minor papilla (b)

the two ducts are dilated. This ectasia is more obvious than the stenosis that may sometimes be difficult to assess (Fig. 65). Furthermore, the prestenotic ectasia is a better criterion for the degree of the stenosis. Even in advanced stenosis the active function can be preserved at least as far as the closing of the sphincter muscle is concerned. Occasionally one can even observe normal papillary motility with its emptying, contraction, and recreation phase (Fig. 66). In such cases, however, the prestenotic ectasia is less obvious. According to the degree of stenosis, the emptying of the pancreatic duct as well as of the common bile duct is delayed. The emptying time can be prolonged up to 15 min or more. The fact that the pancreatic duct is generally emptied before the bile duct may be explained by the smaller quantities of dye needed for opacification of Wirsung's duct. In view of the higher intraductal pressure of the pancreatic duct a potential pancreo-biliary reflux in papillary stenosis cannot be ruled out.

If the stenosis involves only the terminal segment of one of the two ducts, the prestenotic ectasia is confined only to the involved duct that shows delayed emptying (Fig. 67a, b). One case of the authors' ERPC studies presented an advanced stenosis of the distal segment of the common bile duct, in which we could not observe direct emptying from the bile duct but only from the pancreatic duct. During the contraction phase, the markedly dilated bile duct presented shallow indentations. There was a linear functional narrowing of the distal segment of Wirsung's duct. In this phase the common segment of

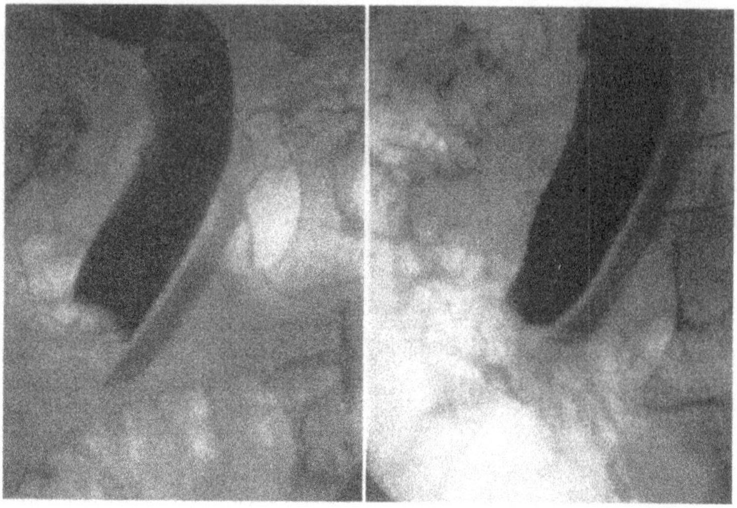

Fig. 68. Hypermotility of papillary duct segments of two ducts. Increased contraction, concave shape of intrapapillary segment of bile duct (a). Following phase (b) shows that concave shape is not due to intrapapillary-wedged concrement

the two duct systems was completely occluded and a small connection between the pancreatic duct and the common bile duct could be observed, suggesting the possibility of a temporary bilio-pancreatic or pancreobiliary reflux mechanism (Fig. 65).

In some papillary stenoses that present the same morphologic signs – such as stenosis of the common segment, prestenotic ectasia of the bile duct, and the pancreatic duct as well as delayed emptying – one can observe a marked hyperperistalsis with increased and prolonged contractions. In such conditions the duodenal peristalsis may occasionally pass over the sphincter contractions as Gomez Oliveros and Rhode (1969) observed. The pronounced contractions can manifest themselves in a bulging of the sphincter muscle and into the lumen of the common bile duct so that the end of the opacified bile duct shows concave contours (Fig. 68). The contours of the narrowed common segment of the two duct systems are smooth and straight. Apparently in such cases the spasm as a functional factor comes to the fore, whereas the other stenoses can be interpreted as secondary to a chronic inflammation with sclerosis, mucosal hyperplasia, adenomyosis, and muscular hypertrophy (Födisch, 1972).

7.5 Benign Tumors of the Pancreas

To date, the number of benign pancreatic tumors detected by ERPC is not remarkable. Safrany (1972a) reports on a case of an islet cell adenoma demonstrated by ERPC; however, since then no other reports of that kind are mentioned in the literature. Doubilet et al. (1959) described a method of peroperative pancreatography for better detection of a tumor of nonductal origin, e.g., of an adenoma. By means of a second injection of contrast material 10 min after the first examination, one can provoke a transitory inflammation of the ductal epithelium and in addition to that an increased permeability of the contrast material with consecutive opacification of the whole parenchyma. This method of demonstrating parenchymal filling defects would be able to detect small lesions situated in the opacified parenchyma. However, since the possible hazards of acinar filling do not allow total opacification of the parenchyma, ERPC cannot be considered a promising method for detection of benign pancreatic tumors.

7.6 Carcinoma of the Pancreas

As soon as ERPC was introduced, numerous investigators examined the diagnostic possibilities for detection of pancreatic carcinoma by the aid of this method (Classen et al., 1972; Hara and Ogoshi, 1973; Belsito et al., 1973; Clouse et al., 1975; Okuda et al., 1973; Robbins et al., 1973; Rohrmann et al., 1973; Stadelmann et al., 1973; Fritsch et al., 1974; Romani et al., 1974; Classen, 1975; Manegold, 1975; Triller

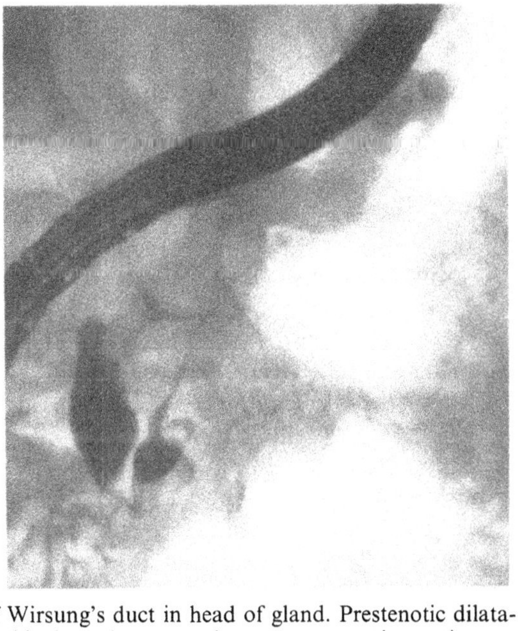

Fig. 69. Irregular stenosis of Wirsung's duct in head of gland. Prestenotic dilatation of main duct and of side branches secondary to pancreatic carcinoma, confirmed by surgery. Due to simultaneous papillary stenosis there is slight dilatation of common bile duct and of poststenotic segment of pancreatic duct. Surgery reveals inoperable tumor. Biopsy was not possible due to severe bleeding

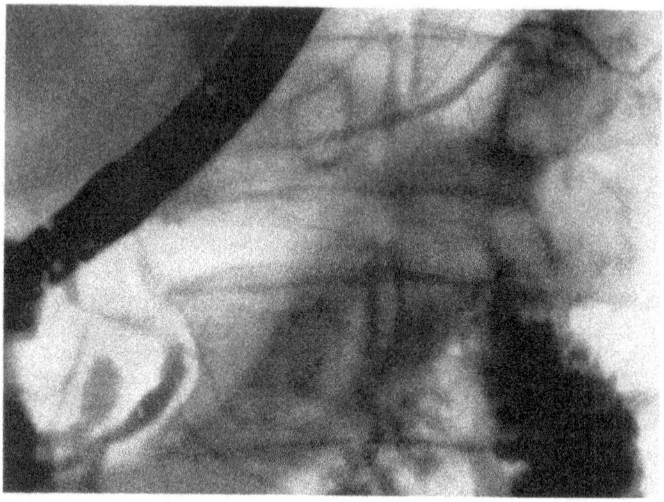

Fig. 70. Irregular stenosis and slight displacement of Wirsung's duct in pancreatic head. Pancreatic carcinoma, confirmed by surgery. Ramus capitis superior, which opens into stenosed segment of main duct, appears hazy and rigid. Absence of prestenotic ectasia of pancreatic duct

et al., 1975; Anacker et al., 1975b). These authors found, that pancreatic carcinoma occurs 2–5 times more often in the head than in the body or the tail. The tail shows the least incidence of pancreatic carcinoma. There is a predominance of the 60–70 age group (Classen, 1972) with males predominating 2 or 3 to 1.

Pancreatic carcinoma can cause the following duct changes:

1. Solitary irregular stenosis with (Fig. 69) or without (Fig. 70) prestenotic ectasia of the main duct.

This sign was already familiar to the investigators who had performed peroperative pancreaticography (Anacker, 1962; Doubilet et al., 1956; Mercadier and Hepp, 1956a; Patel and Lataste, 1954). The authors saw this sign in 17 cases of 47 carcinomas.

2. Occlusion of the main duct.The duct can be abruptly occluded (Fig. 71a), the stop can be hazy (Fig. 71b) or it can be situated at the end of a constantly narrowed segment (tapęred stenosis). Sometimes one can observe several destroyed side branches in the vicinity of the occlusion (Fig. 74). Stenoses combined with prestenotic ectasia and occlusion of the main duct are the most frequent features in carcinoma. Both symptomes have been described by all authors.

The condition of the poststenotic downstream segment of Wirsung's duct is of special diagnostic importance. As a rule, in carcinoma the duct segment between the papilla and the stenosis or occlusion does not show pathologic changes (Figs. 71–74). This finding is in distinct contrast to the changes observed in chronic pancreatitis. When stenosis occurs in chronic pancreatitis, the duct system presents widely spread pathologic changes with ectatic dilatation that can be seen, too, in

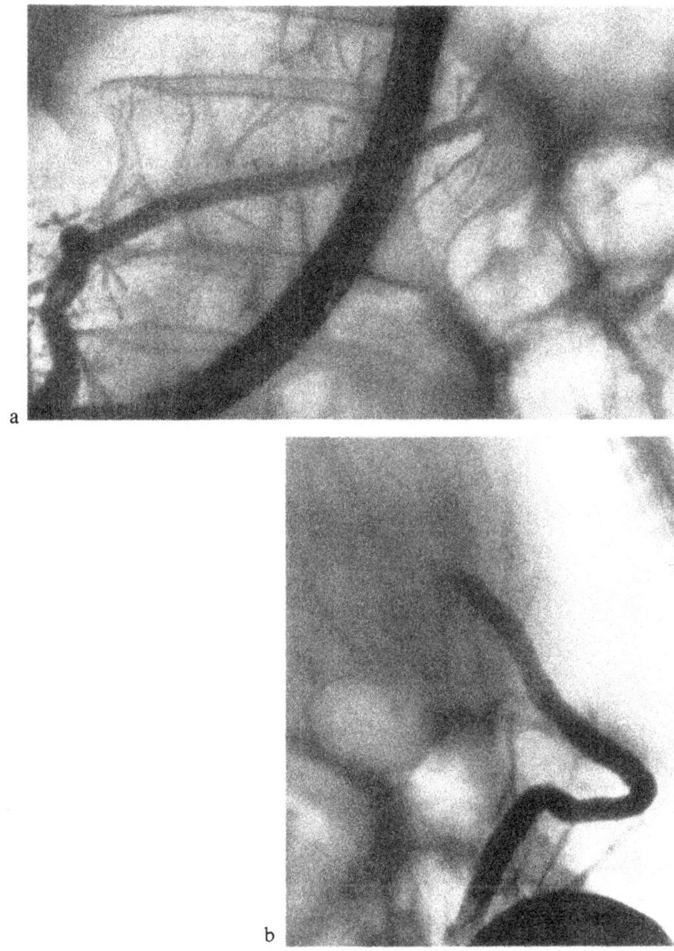

Fig. 71a and b. Complete occlusion of pancreatic main duct in body gland. Occlusion is sharp without tapering as can be seen on lateral roentgenogram (a). Remnant duct system from papilla to occlusion is completely normal (b). Surgery revealed tumor in pancreatic tail the size of child's fist. Histologically confirmed solid carcinoma, with metastases to liver

the poststenotic segments downstream from the stenosis (Fig. 45). This is an important diagnostic criterion. In pancreatic carcinoma the poststenotic segment of Wirsung's duct may only be dilated if papillary evacuation if impaired. However, in such a condition the additional dilatation of the bile duct, which can often be observed, can aid in the diagnosis of papillary stenosis. Of the authors' case material of 47 carcinomas, they observed only two cases with additional papillary stenosis (Fig. 69).

3. Displacement of Wirsung's duct. This finding is rather rare so that few cases are mentioned in the literature (Fig. 75a, b, c). The

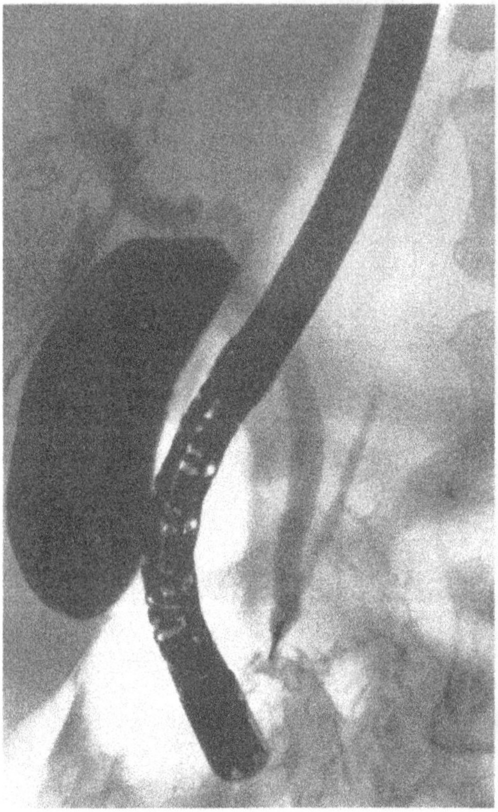

Fig. 72

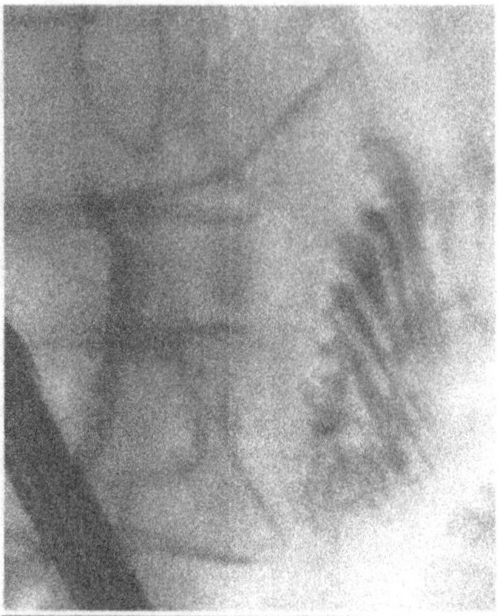

Fig. 73

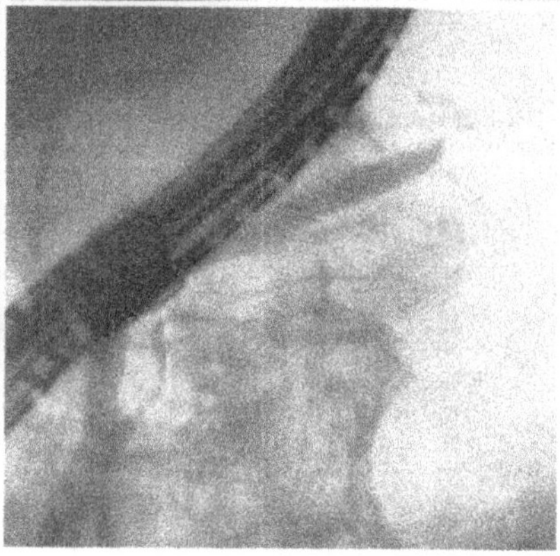

Fig. 74

Fig. 72. Occlusion of Wirsung's duct with hazy contours due to operable carcinoma of pancreatic head 3 cm in size

Fig. 73. Filiform stenosis of Wirsung's duct with slight marginal irregularities in carcinoma of pancreatic body

Fig. 74. Destruction of the side branches in immediate vicinity of highly stenosed Wirsung's duct in pancreatic carcinoma

authors agree with Stadelmann et al. (1972) who consider localized stenosis and occlusion of the main duct combined with displacement as the most characteristic feature of pancreatic carcinoma.

4. Changes of the side branches in the vicinity of the tumor. If the rami and ductuli pancreatici in the neighborhood of the cancer can be visualized which may sometimes be impossible due to technical or pathoanatomical reasons, they may give additional information. One can observe cystic destruction, fragmentation, displacement, and rarefication. A pancreaticogram that presents cystic changes of the small side branches in the vicinity of the tumor combined with stenosis

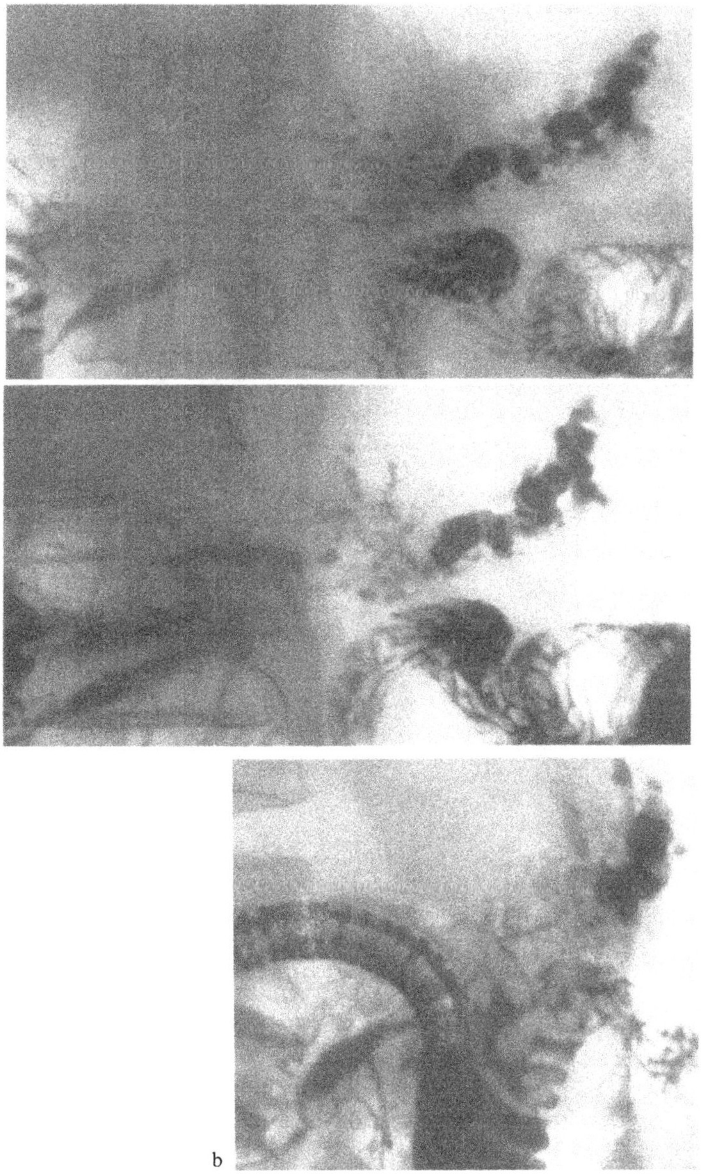

a

c

b

Fig. 75. Irregular stenosis and arciform displacement (*b*) of pancreatic main duct in surgically confirmed pancreatic carcinoma. Cystic distraction and fragmentation of rami and ductuli in vicinity of tumor (*c*). Prestenotic dilatation of pancreatic head. Area of destroyed duct system indicates size of tumor (*a*). At surgery inoperable tumor of pancreatic head was found. Encasement of common bile duct and metastases to lymphnodes

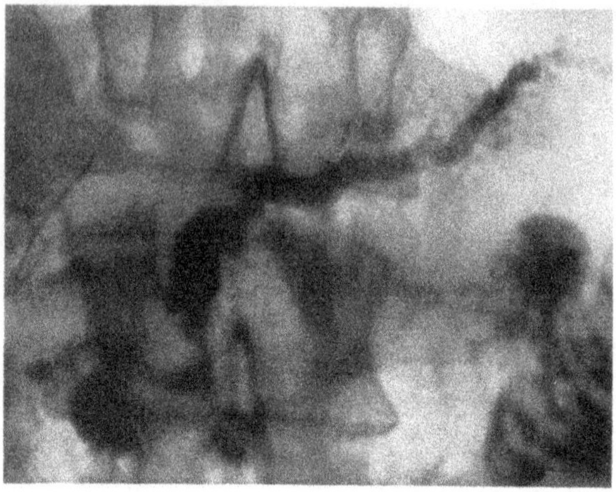

a

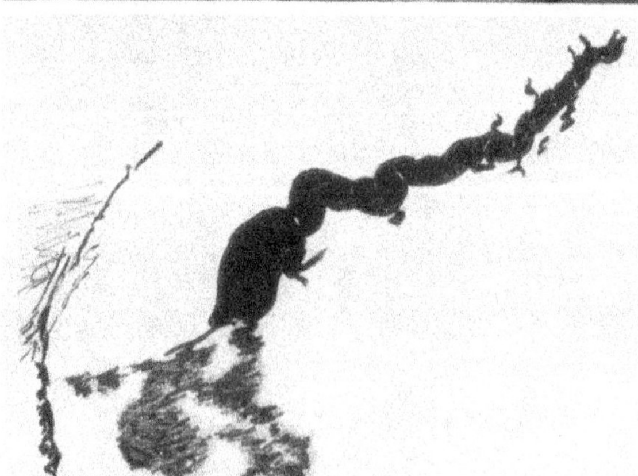

b

Fig. 76a and b. Stenosis of Wirsung's duct in head of gland. Prestenotic ectasia in carcinoma of pancreatic head. Multiple irregular lacunary pools in necrotic cavity of tumor

or occlusion of the main duct, corresponds largely to the pathologic-anatomical pattern of a cystadenoma.

5. Lacunary pooling of contrast material. In about one-fifth of all cases of pancreatic carcinoma one can observe lacunary pooling of contrast material as a sign of tumor destruction (Figs. 76a, b). These pools are usually found to be multiple with irregular hazy contours. On technical grounds they often cannot be distinguished from lacunary pools secondary to a peptic process and to pseudocysts (Stender et al., 1974). However, when judging those changes, one should always consider the gneral radiographic picture of the pancreaticogram (Figs. 77a, b).

6. Changes of the common bile duct. Stenosis of the common bile duct is a rather frequent concomitant sign not only of chronic pancreatitis but also of pancreatic carcinoma (Oi et al., 1970; Classen et al.,

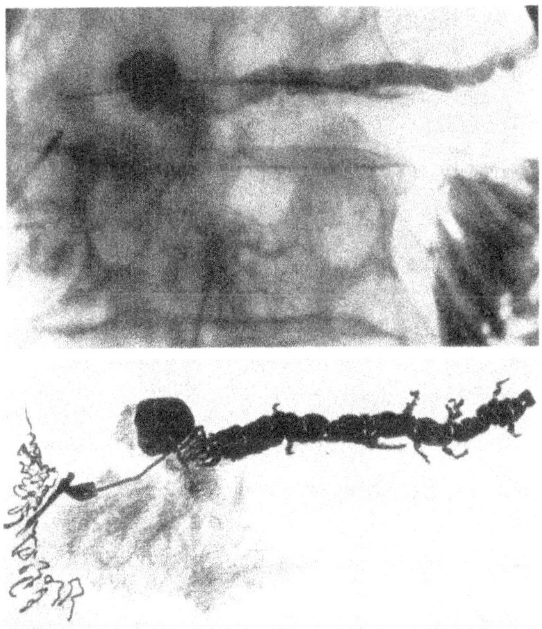

Fig. 77a and b. Hair-thin stenosis of Wirsung's duct in pancreatic head with prestenotic dilatation and multiple necrotic cavities not clearly separated from one another. At surgery tumor 5 × 5 cm was found in pancreatic head. Frozen sections revealed pancreatic carcinoma. Encasement of portal vein, of middle colic artery, and of superior mesenteric artery. Metastases to regional lymphnodes

1972; Robbins et al., 1973; Stadelmann et al., 1973; and Zeus, 1973). This is due to the predominant incidence of carcinoma in the pancreatic head. It would surely be found more often if simultaneous visualization of the bile duct could constantly be realized in ERPC. If the stenosis has smooth borders, the aspect of the common bile duct alone does not give information as to the nature of the constriction (Fig. 78). An irregular contour of the narrowed section of the bile duct is indicative of malignant tumor invasion; the distance between the occlusion of the pancreatic duct and the bile duct allows us to assess the size of the tumor (Figs. 79, 80). Sometimes there may be calculi in the blocked biliary tract in the hepatic ducts or in the gallbladder (Figs. 72, 78). If the stenosis of the retropancreatic segment of the common bile duct is the only pathologic findings, for example in cases in which retrograde filling of the pancreatic ducts fails, the presence of a primary carcinoma of the bile duct cannot be excluded.

Classification of Pancreatic Carcinoma in ERPC. ERPC allows us to coordinate the carcinoma to the anatomicpathologic conditions that are determined by the site of tumor formation within the gland. The carcinoma develops from the ducts or from the epithelium of the acini

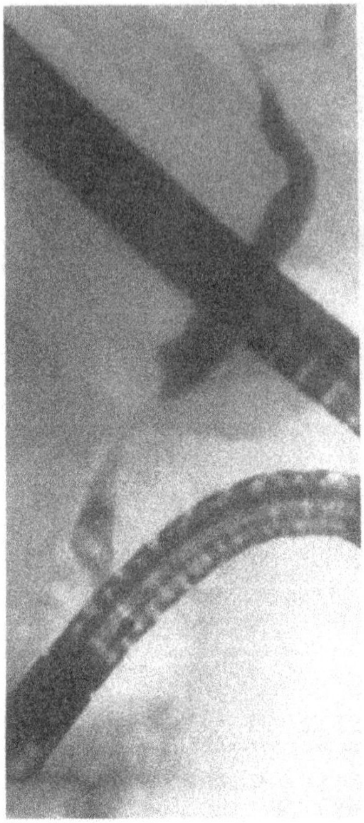

Fig. 78

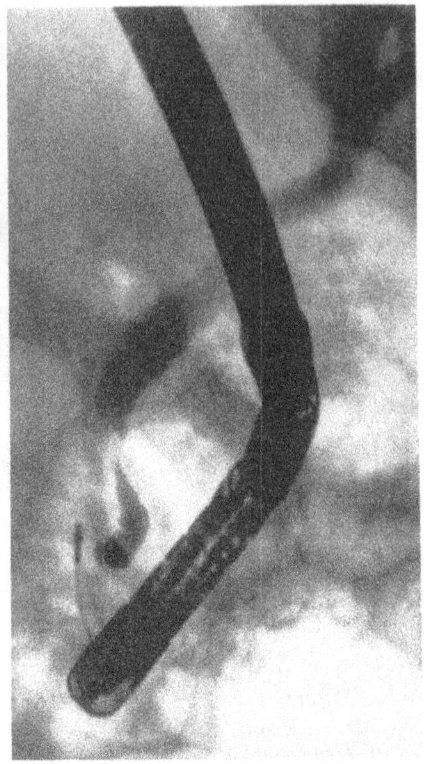

Fig. 79

Fig. 78. Smooth annular stenosis of common bile duct in pancreatic carcinoma. Multiple concrements in prepapillary segment of common bile duct. Postmortem examination revealed tumor of size of plum in head of gland

Fig. 79. Stenosis of common bile duct presenting marginal irregularities. Prestenotic dilatation in pancreatic carcinoma

(Becker, 1973). According to this, one can differentiate two different types of carcinoma in the pancreaticogram (Mercadier and Hepp, 1956a; Anacker, 1962; Hara and Ogoshi, 1973):

I. The canalicular carcinoma arising from the duct system.

a) Carcinoma arising from the main duct. Here the main duct, Wirsung's duct or Santorini's duct is mostly occluded and eventually destroyed. In the very neighborhood of the tumor, the side branches are destroyed or deformed. The authors found these roentgen features in 15 out of 47 cases.

b) Carcinoma arising from the side branches. This pattern is characterized by cystic ectasia, fragmentation, or deformation of the rami pancreatici in the tumor region. The main duct is narrowed and shows characteristic displacement. This picture corresponds histologically to the cystadenocarcinoma. The authors observed it in 6 of 47 cases.

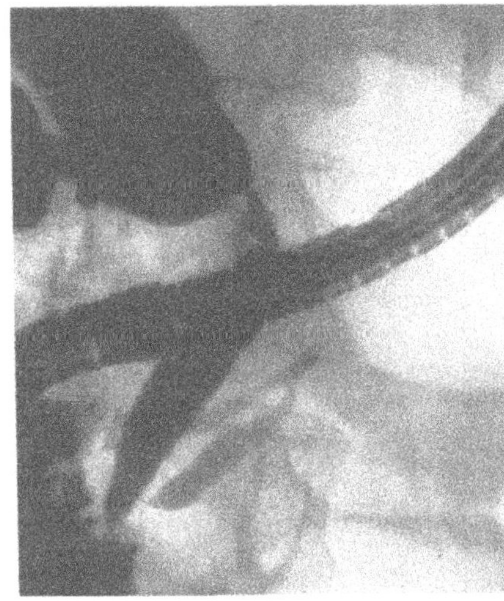

Fig. 80. Pancreatic carcinoma with occlusion of Wirsung's duct. Irregular stenosis of common bile duct with marked prestenotic dilatation. Distance between occlusion of pancreatic duct and stenosis of bile duct indicates minimal size of tumor. Surgery revealed inoperable tumor

II. Carcinoma arising from the epithelium of the acini.

a) In this pattern displacement of the main duct, which may be narrowed, is well anterior. Major side branches are rigid due to tumor encasement. Considering the anatomical picture, one may expect occlusion of the smaller branches of the ductuli and canaliculi and therewith rarefication of the draining ducts in the tumor region. The carcinoma arising from the epithelium of the acini is much less frequent than the carcinoma of ductal origin (Becker, 1973). Of 47 cases the authors observed it in only 2 patients. Hara and Ogoshi (1973) report on 4 of 21 cases. The authors observed the same roentgenographic features in a case of multiple metastases to the gland.

b. Completely different duct changes are caused by the myxocarcinoma. In this tumor the viscous, gelatin-like mucus produced by the tumor glands is gradually transported into the duct system until it fills and blocks the main duct as well as the side branches proximal and distal to the carcinoma. The roentgenographic picture obtained by filling of the ducts with contrast material is so grotesque that the original pattern of the former duct system can hardly be recognized (Fig. 81 a, b). Instead of the well-organized duct system there is a variety of diverticulalike lacunary pools communicating with completely irregular draining ducts. A postmortem study on a resected specimen shows that this marked, irregular ectasia cannot be secondary to a tumor stenosis. The opacified poststenotic duct segment downstream from the tumor shows an enormous dilatation and irregular course whereas the papillary passage is not blocked. It is the gelatin-like viscous mucus

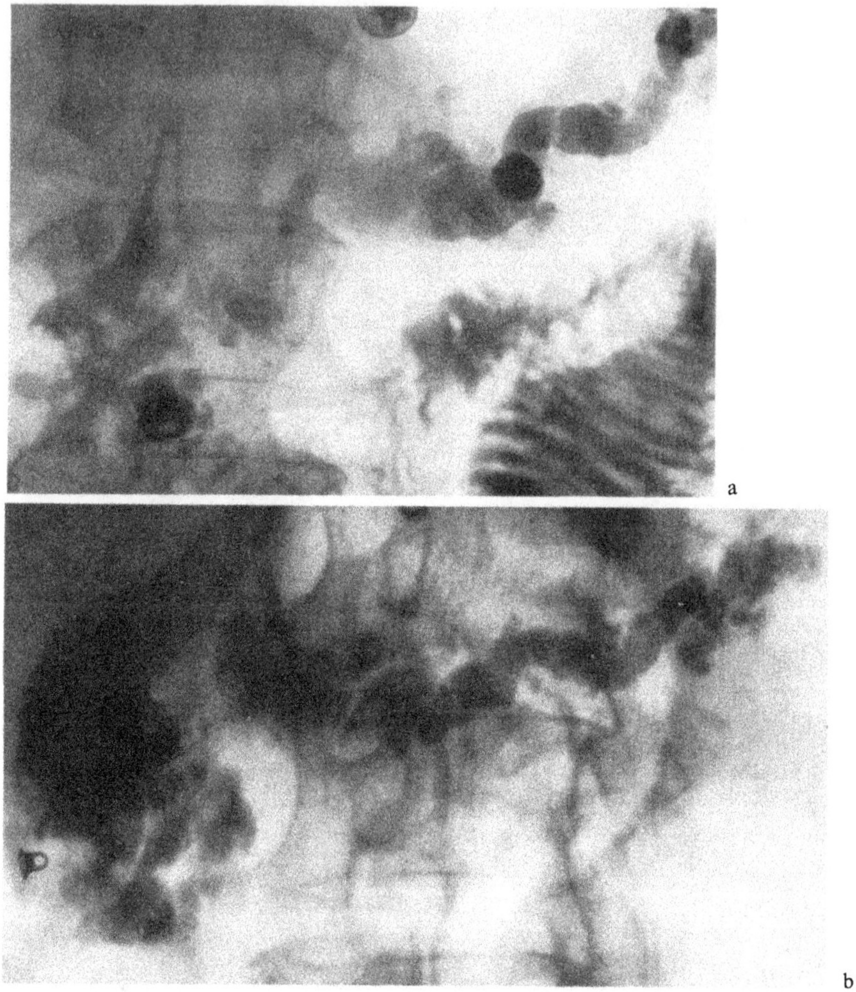

Fig. 81 a and b. Cystic destructions of side branches in pancreatic head (a). Further filling revealed grotesque ectasia of entire duct system mainly in isthmus and in head of gland (b). This aspect is strongly suggestive of myxocarcinoma. Surgery revealed ragged tumor of fist size in pancreatic head. Tumor encasement of bile duct

stuffed constantly into the duct system that must be considered as the cause of the heavy deformations of the whole duct system. Compared to this mechanism, the immediate tumor deformations that the gland undergoes are of minor importance. In the outlined case, the head of the gland had reached the size of a fist whereas the tumor did not exceed the size of a cherry. These findings corroborate the repeated observation that pancreatic carcinoma can be embedded in an inflammatory swelling of the gland. This is particularly true in carcinomas that have occluded the duct. For these reasons peroperative diagnosis, even when supported by exploratory excision and histologic examination, can encounter difficulties. In the myxocarcinoma it is the mucus that hinders the flow of pancreatic juice, producing by this mechanism the heavy pathologic changes with serious sequelae of infection, necrosis, fibrotic healing process, and indurations.

Thus, in pancreatic carcinoma, in canalicular, and myxocarcinoma, one can find the same sequelae as can be seen in chronic relapsing pancreatitis secondary to stenosis of the duct. The last-mentioned case of myxo-carcinoma may be an example of such sequelae. In addition to the monstrous ectasia of the ducts, the head and the tail of the gland were enlarged to double their normal size and interspersed with multiple calcifications. Upstream from the stenosis was a pyoid abscess. In the tail the normal parenchyma was substituted by fatty tissue and the ducts were obliterated (Fig. 81 a, b).

A better understanding of clinical symptoms and exact planning of surgical intervention are facilitated by classification of pancreatic carcinomas into two basic forms according to their site of origin with regard to the fact that transitional forms are possible. The canalicular carcinoma of type I, while causing early occlusion of the main duct, leads to early symptoms of excretory insufficiency unless the second main duct communicates with the duodenum. In contrast to this, the carcinoma arising from the acini does not lead to excretory disorders over a long period of growth as long as the main duct is not involved. Involvement of the common bile duct, which is independent of the nature of the cancer, is determined by the site of the tumor, i.e., whether it is situated in the pancreatic head or not.

In carcinoma the diagnostic accuracy of ERPC (Table 5) may be judged as good in view of the early involvement of the main duct and the predominance of type I.

Table 5. Diagnostic *accuracy of ERPC* in pancreatic carcinoma

	No. of cases	Correct diagnosis	False	
			positive	negative
Survey of the literature by Romani (1974)	153	95%	–	–
Authors' case material (1975)	47	91%	4%	4%

The occasional failure in visualization of the pancreatic duct, partly due to technical reasons (Classen et al., 1972) and partly secondary to tumor invasion of the papilla (Belsito et al., 1973; and Burwood et al., 1973) detracts from this method. Diagnostic accuracy is improved by aspiration of juice for cytologic examination (Kozu, 1973; Witte, 1973; Endo et al., 1974; Hatfield et al., 1974). More accurate cytologic results may be obtained by abrasive brush biopsy of the duct system, a method introduced by Weidenhiller et al. (1975). Of 25 patients, sufficient cytologic material could be obtained in 19 cases from the pancreatic duct and in 6 cases from the common bile duct. In one patient preoperative diagnosis could be established with certainty by cytologic study, while by means of ERPC alone pancreatic cancer could only be suspected.

The differential diagnosis of pancreatic carcinoma in ERPC can only be established by considering the whole roentgenographic pattern. Isolated symptoms detached from the other features as irregular solitary stenosis, prestenotic ectasia, displacement of the main duct, and lacunary pooling can be observed also in chronic pancreatitis and pancreatic necrosis. However, in chronic pancreatitis these signs are always combined with general deformations of the whole duct system, especially of the smaller branches (Figs. 45–48), whereas in carcinoma these changes can only be demonstrated in the prestenotic duct section (Figs. 75–77). On the other hand, when diagnosing pancreatic carcinoma, one must take into consideration each of the other individual signs mentioned above. Here the normal shape of the poststenotic segment of the main duct can be particularly helpful for differential diagnosis (Figs. 71–73, 75). In 1974 Nette reported on different criteria for differential diagnosis of changes of the small branches in chronic pancreatitis and in pancreatic carcinoma: Whereas in chronic pancreatitis the ectasia involves all segments of the small branches, in carcinoma the distal segments of the branches are of normal width. The authors' case material could not confirm this observation in all cases. For differentiation of pancreatitis and pancreatic carcinoma, Belsito et al. (1973) have studied the emptying time of the prestenotic dilated duct. In all 16 of his pancreatic carcinoma he found a delayed emptying time of at least 20 min cases, whereas in chronic pancreatitis the duct system had emptied within normal limits. The authors could not confirm this latter observation in all inflammatory dilatations; on the other hand, they observed normal emptying time in ducts occluded by pancreatic carcinoma. For these reasons they feel that this sign should be judged with caution. It goes without saying that for establishing a differential diagnosis, all other roentgenologic and clinical findings should be combined with the findings in ERPC.

When reviewing the role of ERPC in the early diagnosis of pancreatic carcinoma the authors admit that up to now, the majority of all carcinomas found by ERPC that have been reported on in the literature as well as of the authors' case material were in an advanced state and only a small minority were operable. However, the possibility of establishing an early diagnosis of pancreatic cancer by means of ERPC cannot be denied as far as the method itself is concerned. This is true at least in those carcinomas that arise from the duct system. As in other malignant tumors, the unchallenged problem is the difficulty of early detection of clinically suspect cases. This may be rather impossible in carcinomas of type II arising from the acini that may remain

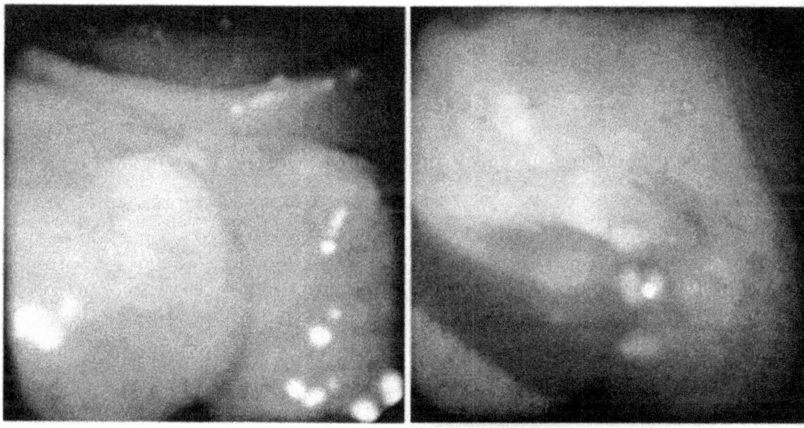

Fig. 82a

b

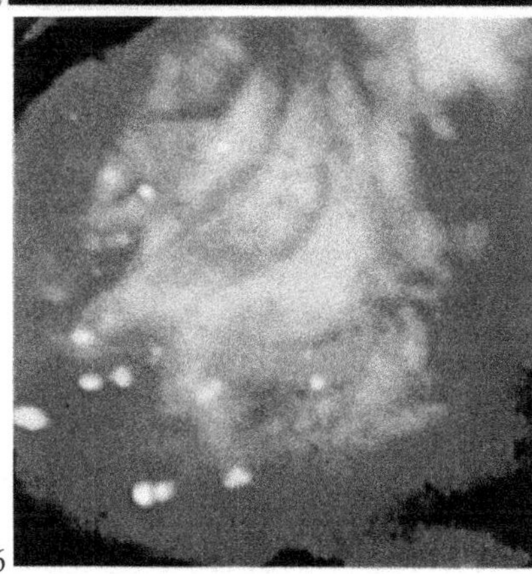

Fig. 86

Fig. 82a and b. Large, ragged, hypervascularized tumor at papilla of Vater protruding into lumen of duodenum (a). Endoscopic forceps biopsy revealed papillary carcinoma

Fig. 86. Endoscopic aspect of tumor encasement of duodenal wall by carcinoma of pancreatic head. Flattening of coarse mucosal folds

clinically unsuspected for a long time. With regard to other tumor types, ERPC and other techniques (above all angiography) should be performed as soon as the first clinical signs arouse suspicion.

7.7 Papillary Carcinoma

Duodenoscopy, while providing a close face-on view of the papilla, enables us to diagnose directly papillary cancer. The carcinoma leads to enlargement and destruction of the papilla, which occasionally protrudes into the lumen of the duodenum like a hypervascularized and ulcerated tumor (Fig. 82a). At the touch of the instrument the tumor easily shows bleeding. The orifice of the papilla is often occluded by the tumor and cannot be cannulated so that ERPC fails. On the other

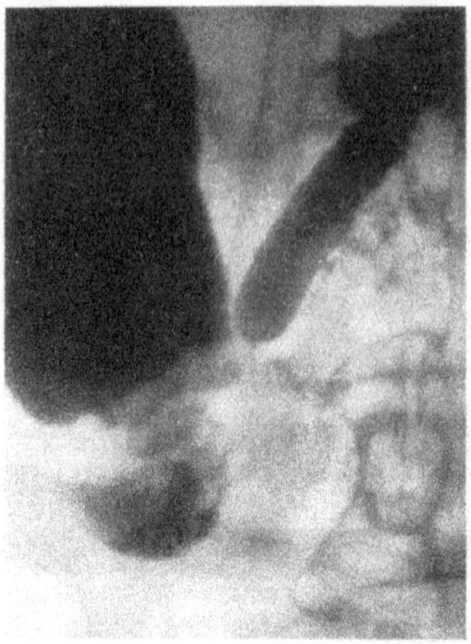

Fig. 83. Irregular stenosis 2.5 cm long as thin as a knitting needle in prepapillary segment of common bile duct. Prestenotic ectasia of entire Wirsung's duct and its side branches. Distinct ectasia of common bile duct, which is 8 times as wide as normal. Endoscopy showed ragged tumor of papilla with contact bleeding. Brush biopsy revealed adenocarcinoma. At surgery walnut-sized tumor was found

hand, the tumor may manifest itself as a shallow crater showing an eroded granular orifice (Oi et al., 1970). The diagnosis is made by exploratory deep biopsy and histologic examination (Fig. 82b).

Thus, duodenoscopy is the method of choice in diagnosis, even in early diagnosis of papillary cancer, in spite of the fact that endoscopy and biopsy cannot detect all cases of papillary cancer (Oi).

As a rule, in successful cannulation one can observe advanced ectasia of the whole duct system and sometimes of the common bile duct, too, secondary to the tumor blockade (Fig. 83). In papillary stenosis and papillary cancer, ectasia and delayed emptying of the ducts correspond to the varying involvement of the pancreatic duct or the biliary duct. Thus one can find in both conditions different ectasia of the two ducts. In the same way emptying of contrast material corresponds to the different involvement of the duct systems. In papillary stenosis secondary to scarring the emptying phase from the dilated pancreatic duct, respectively from the dilated bile duct is considerably delayed in papillary cancer, too.

In successful cannulation of the orifice the intraductal part of the tumor can be demonstrated as a filling defect in the pancreatic duct or in the bile duct (Sobbe et al., 1975) (Fig. 84a, b). As the authors observed in one case, ectasia does not always show the degree expected (Fig. 85).

When the tumor involves the neighboring part of the gland rather than the papilla, it usually cannot be differentiated from pancreatic carcinoma of the head, either radiologically nor by gross or microscopic

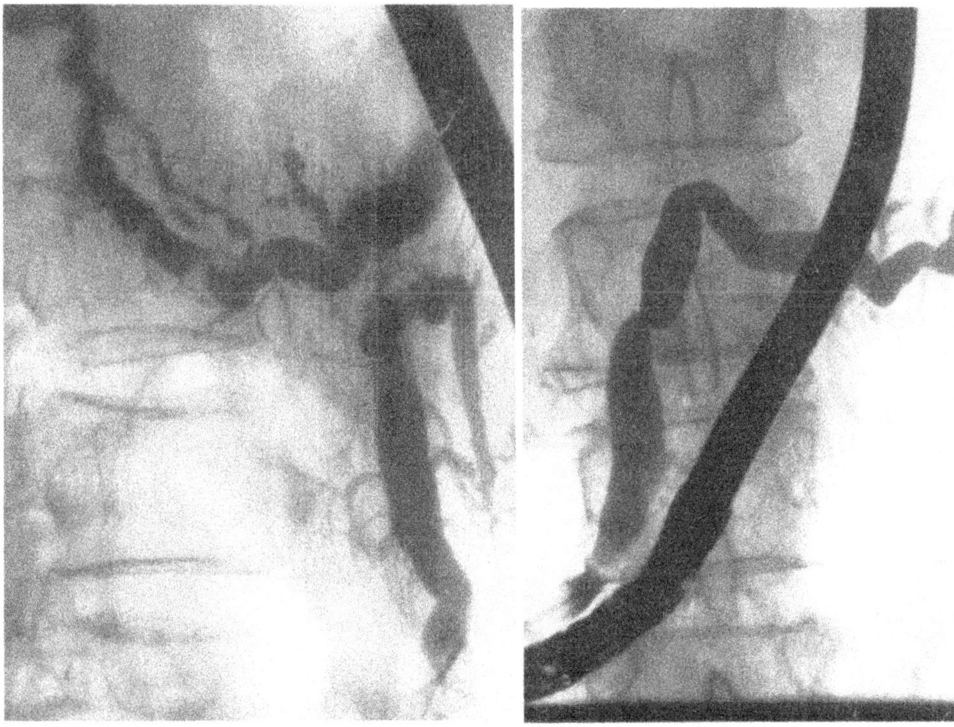

a b

Fig. 84a and b. Papillary carcinoma. A 4-mm long part of tumor has proliferated into pancreatic duct and leads to prestenotic ectasia of entire duct system. Detailed pictures demonstrate intraductal part of neoplasm. Brush biopsy revealed adenocarcinoma

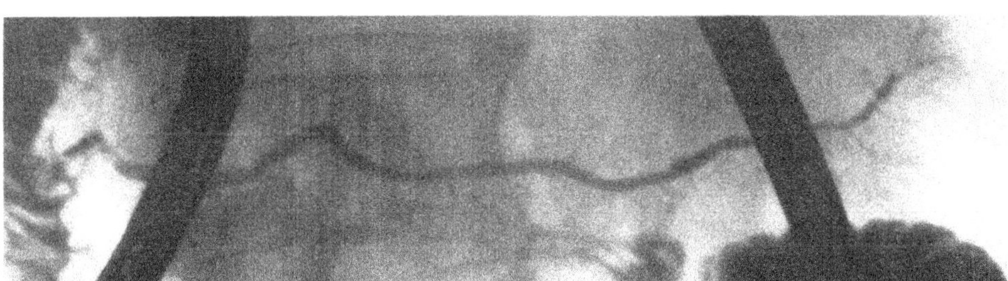

Fig. 85. Papillary carcinoma confirmed by endoscopic biopsy. Cannulation was successful. Small part of tumor manifests itself as filling defect in very prepapillary segment. Absence of ectasia proximal to tumor

Fig. 86 see p. 91

features. Tumor invasion into the duodenal wall can be seen endoscopically; however, it is not confined to the papilla but extends into the neighboring area (Fig. 86). Thus, pancreatic cancer invading the duodenal wall cannot be excluded. Cannulation is often feasible; the roentge-

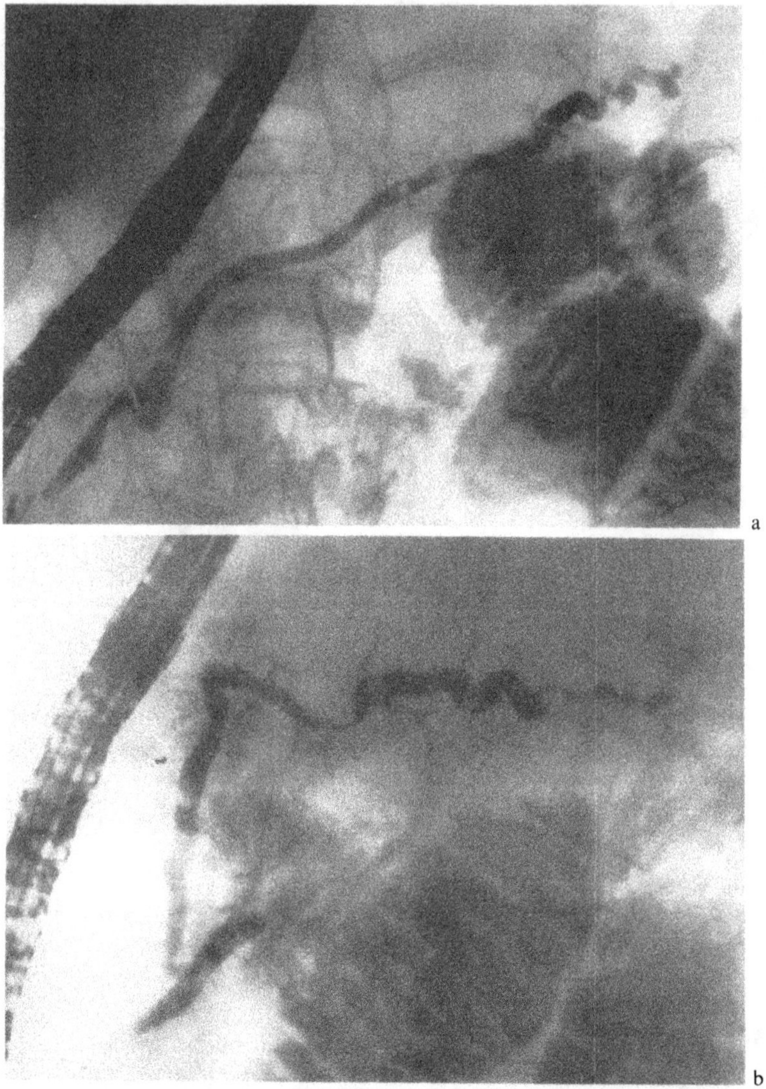

Fig. 87a and b. Metastases to pancreas in patient with hypernephroma. Multiple metastases throughout abdomen. Slight displacement and narrowing of pancreatic duct in head and in tail (a). Distinct backward displacement of entire pancreatic tail (b)

nographic features do not differ from those of pancreatic carcinoma close to the papilla.

7.8 Metastases of Tumors to the Pancreas

The authors had the opportunity to observe a patient who presented with metastases of a tumor to the pancreas. The 58-year-old woman

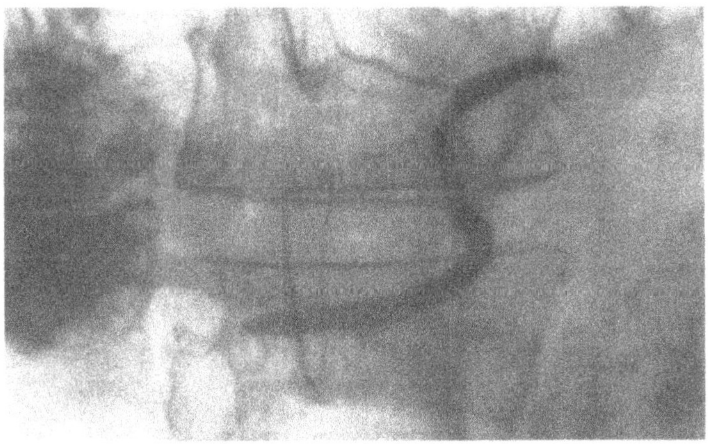

Fig. 88. Patient with pancreaticojejunostomy. Good draining function of anastomosis with emptying of contrast material into jejunum

had been subjected to nephrectomy of the left kidney for hypernephroma. Five years later arteriography revealed a hypernephroma of the right kidney with multiple metastases to the abdomen. ERPC showed circumscribed displacement and slight stenosis of the pancreatic duct at two distant segments, one in the head and the other in the tail (Fig. 87a). A slight ectasia could be observed only proximal to the stenosis in the tail. There was considerable backward displacement of the entire pancreatic duct (Fig. 87b).

7.9 Posttraumatic Conditions of the Pancreas

As a result of an injury with consecutive lesion of the pancreatic duct, the trauma may lead to formation of a pseudocyst in the same way as in postnecrotic peptic liquefaction. In such an event the gland often presents the picture of so-called posttraumatic pancreatitis. Up to now there are no reports on such cases studied by ERPC. One might expect duct changes as in chronic pancreatitis combined with signs of pseudocyst formation, and above all escape of contrast material from the affected duct.

7.10 Postoperative Conditions of the Pancreas

ERPC is especially qualified for postoperative studies after surgical intervention on the duct system, above all in anastomoses of the ducts with the gastrointestinal tract. The potency of a pancreaticojejunostomy can be checked by documentation of the dye escaping from the duct into the jejunum (Fig. 88). At the same time the condition of the remaining duct system and an eventual improvement of the changes preoperatively documentated can be assessed. Proper caution should be exercised in indicating ERPC in patients with previous sphincter surgery. ERPC with cannulation of the sphincter of Oddi, following a very delicate

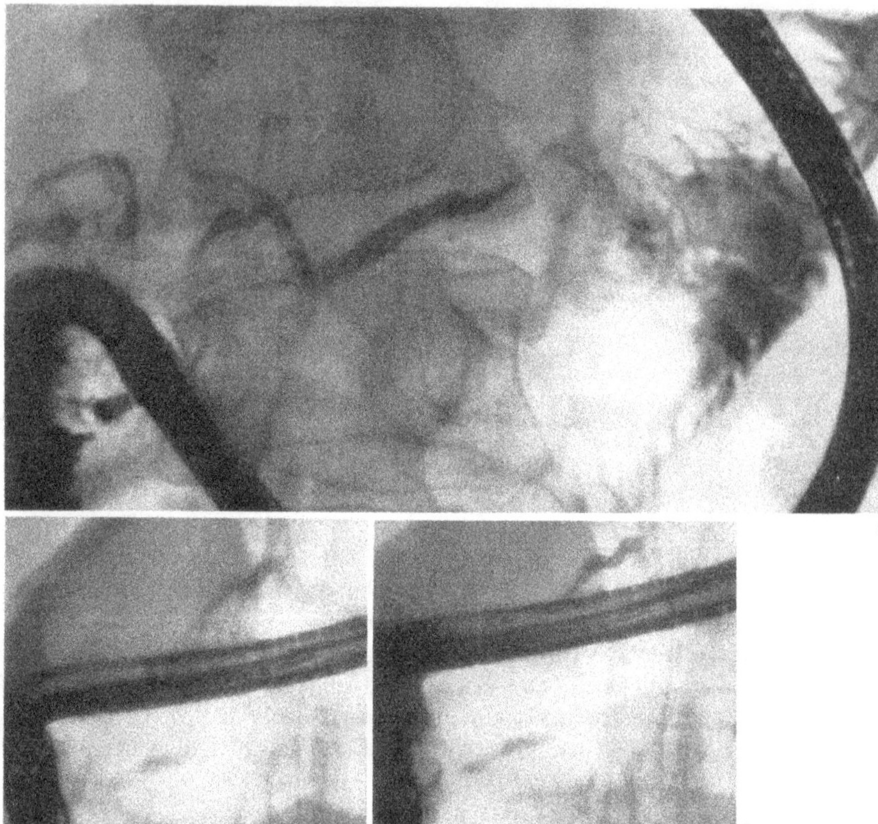

Fig. 89a and b. Patient with papillotomy and pancreaticojejunostomy. Good draining function of papilla and anastomosis. Distinct emptying of contrast material into duodenum and jejunum (a). Papilla shows an emptying phase (right) and retraction phase (left)

operation such as sphincterotomy or sphincteroplasty, does not seem to be advisable. Furthermore, in postoperative conditions the mechanical irritation of the papilla due to cannulation does not allow a precise assessment of the emptying mechanism. Such a control may only be indicated in the later postoperative phase several weeks after operation (Fig. 89a, b).

As far as anastomoses of the biliary tract to the bowel are concerned, ERPC is well indicated in choledochojejunostomy as it provides a good function control (Miederer et al., 1974). As a rule, in this condition one cannot visualize the anastomosis by upper gastrointestinal barium studies even if the patient is carefully positioned. The condition of a choledochoduodenostomy, however, can easily and adequately be checked by barium studies.

8. ERPC in Diseases of the Biliary Tract

Successful visualization of the biliary tree can be obtained by endoscopic retrograde cholangiography in 74%. Up to now the exact cause of occasional failure of simultaneous filling of the two duct systems remains unknown. Since the biliary sphincter is stronger than the sphincter of the pancreatic duct, contraction or spasm of the sphincter muscle is incriminated. To date there is no reliable technique for constant reproducible retrograde filling of the bile ducts. For this reason the other techniques of cholangiography, including percutaneous transhepatic cholangiography, are sometimes indispensable when retrograde cholangiography fails.

8.1 Primary Sclerosing Cholangitis

Primary sclerosing cholangitis is a rare disease of unknown origin characterized histologically by diffuse proliferation of fibrous tissue surrounding the biliary ducts. The extrahepatic ducts are constantly involved, the intrahepatic ducts are occasionally affected. Primary sclerosing cholangitis develops spontaneously, and it can be associated with ulcerative colitis, granulomatous colitis (Crohn's disease), sclerosing mediastinitis, retroperitoneal fibrosis, and orbital pseudotumors. ERPC reveals the following roentgenographic features (Geisse, 1973; Classen and Demling, 1973):

As a rule, the common bile duct and often some intrahepatic ducts are narrowed (Fig. 90). The common bile duct is rarely spared. In a widely spread involvement of the intrahepatic bile ducts, when retrograde filling only visualizes major branches with stenoses and variations in caliber, this condition presents the aspect of "pruning" of branches.

Since retrograde cholangiography often fails for the reasons mentioned above, one must draw on percutaneous transhepatic cholangiography for precise demonstration of the biliary tract (Geisse et al., 1973).

8.2 Secondary Sclerosing Cholangitis and Postoperative Conditions of the Biliary Tract

Secondary sclerosing cholangitis is defined as proliferation of fibrous tissue around the bile ducts secondary to a previous surgical intervention on the upper abdomen, especially on the bile ducts (Geisse et al., 1973). ERPC is indicated in postoperative cholostasis when the serum

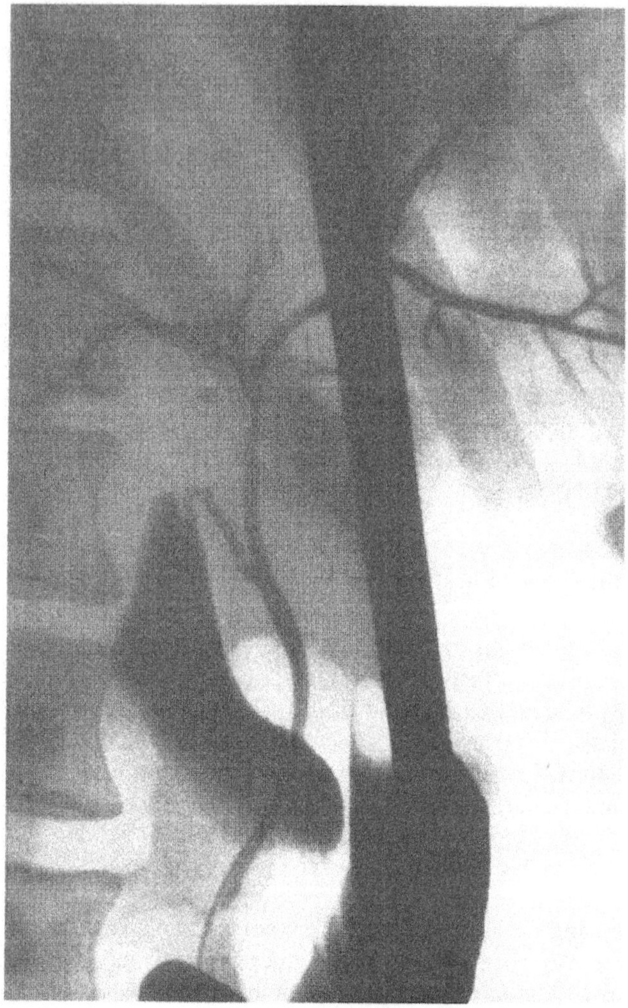

Fig. 90. Circumscribed stenosis at medial wall of common bile duct, immediately distal to branching of right hepatic and left hepatic duct. Slight marginal irregularities. Remnant duct system is completely normal. Aspect suggests primary sclerosing cholangitis

bilirubin level exceeds 4 mg % with consecutive negative result in orthodox cholangiography (Sobbe et al., 1975).

The ERPC roentgenographic pattern is similar to that found in primary sclerosing cholangitis (Fig. 29), except that the predominant stenosis is found at the junction of the hepatic duct and the common bile duct in the neighborhood of the former cholecystectomy. Here, when the cystic duct inosculates with the bile ducts, one often finds a solitary stenosis secondary to cholecystectomy.

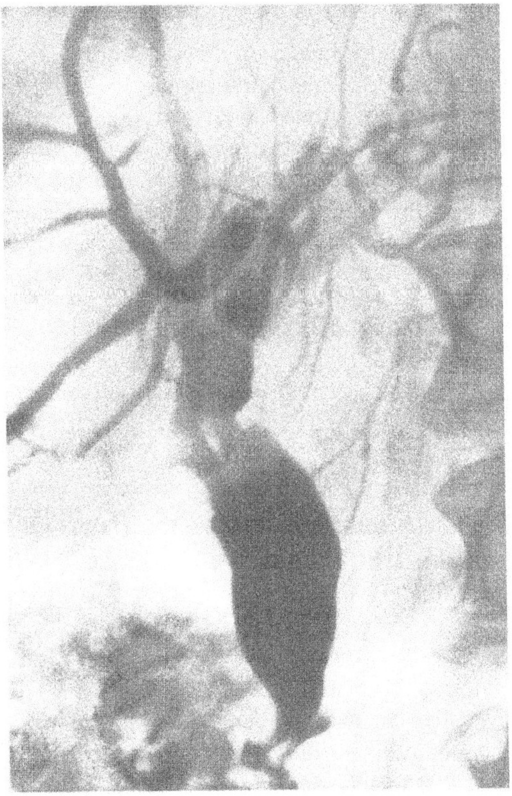

Fig. 91. Retrograde cholangiography. Patient had previously been subjected to cholecystectomy on behalf of calculous disease. Endoscopy shows duodenal fistula (perforation of concrement). After cannulation of fistula, common bile duct and hepatic duct were filled. At junction of fistula common bile duct is drawn laterally near duodenum and slightly narrowed. Marked dilatation of common bile duct and hepatic duct in papillary stenosis. Short retrograde reflux from bile duct into pancreatic duct, via ampulla of Vater

According to George (1973) and Way and Sleisinger (1973) 95% benign stenoses are secondary to surgical intervention. Occasionally the stricture, which can be secondary as well to choledochoduodenostomy, may reach such an extent prestenotic bile ducts can be widened. Especially in marked stenoses, retrograde filling often visualizes only the distal part of the duct; the contrast material does not pass beyond the stenosis. However, as the extent of the stenosis should be assessed preoperatively, additional information must be supplied by other cholangiographic methods. On the other hand, in view of the potential risk of septic cholangitis following ERPC, attempts at complete filling of the ducts beyond the stenosis may not be advisable. T-tube cholangiography performed in the postoperative phase cannot exclude a stricture due to secondary sclerosing cholangitis, for the stenosis develops only after a longer interval.

The authors observed a patient presenting a fistula between the common bile duct and the descending duodenum. Cholecystectomy had been performed some years before because of calculi in the gallbladder. Endoscopy revealed a fistula-like opening in the descending duodenum that was easy to cannulate. Retrograde filling visualized the markedly widened common bile duct and the radicals of the hepatic duct. At the junction of the cystic duct there was a relative narrowing. The common bile duct was drawn close to the opening of the fistula revealing a conical shape. The papilla of Vater was found 2 cm distal to the fistula. There was a short reflux of dye from the common bile duct into the main duct (Fig. 91).

ERPC is an appropriate diagnostic technique, not only for detecting strictures of the bile duct but also for visualization of postoperative fistulae and lesions with coexistent pericholecystic abscess.

8.3 Calculous Disease of the Bile Ducts and the Gallbladder

Demonstration of calculi in the bile ducts and the gallbladder by means of ERPC is much more reliable than by aid of peroral or transvenous cholangiography (Fig. 92). However, the bile ducts may sometimes be overfilled so that the contours of the calculi may be concealed by the opaque contrast material. In such conditions Stadelmann et al. (1973), and Classen and Demling (1973) propose to let the bile ducts empty and to repeat filling taking spot films under television control and if necessary using the compression cone as in orthodox cholangiography.

In order to establish a reliable diagnosis of calculous disease of the biliary tract after filling of the ducts and retracting of the instrument, the roentgenographic study of bile ducts and gallbladder should be performed in the usual way in upright and recumbent positions as in excretory cholangiography.

One can often observe stones in the common bile duct proximal to a stenosis secondary to pancreatic carcinoma (Fig. 78).

The differential diagnosis of calculous disease of the common bile duct must take into consideration coagulated blood and biliary gravel. Calculi are characterized by localized filling defects and sometimes by facet contours. In papillary spasm during the retraction phase, the sphincter muscle can bulge into the lumen of the slightly dilated common bile duct imitating the picture of a solitary concrement (Fig. 68). The correct diagnosis can be made by studying the emptying phase (Anacker et al., 1973).

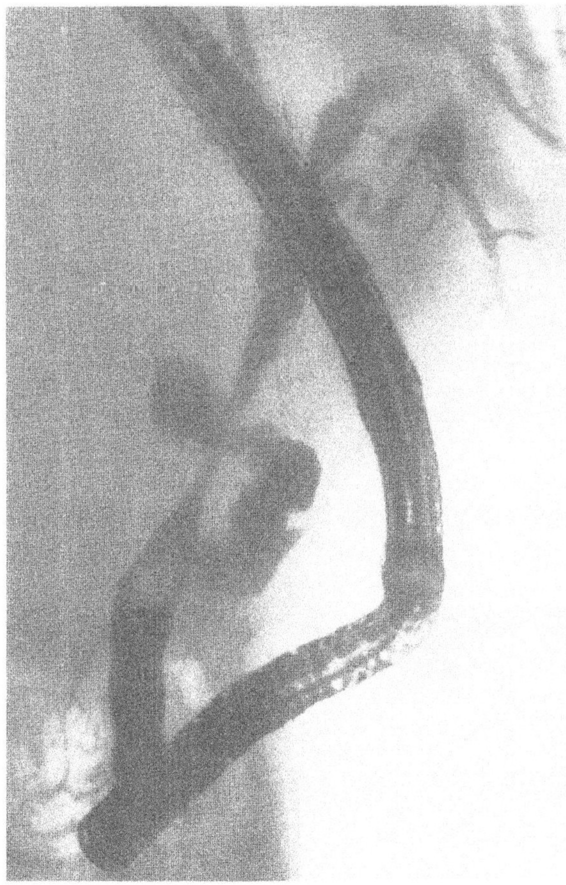

Fig. 92. Carcinoma of biliary tract with tubular stenosis of hepatic duct and prestenotic ectasia of intrahepatic segments of biliary tree. Ectasia of common bile duct and cystic duct with solitary concrement in common bile duct

8.4 Carcinoma of the Bile Ducts and Carcinoma of the Liver

Several authors have reported on carcinoma of the biliary tree detected by ERPC (Robbins, 1973; Geisse et al., 1975; and Sobbe et al., 1975). One can often find a localized stenosis combined with marginal irregularities frequently situated in the proximal segment of the common bile duct (Fig. 92). A predominant localization is the junction of the left and right branches of the hepatic duct. The stenosis is some centimenters long and extends to the common hepatic duct. The segments proximal to the stenosis – the right and left main biliary ducts – are dilated. Sometimes there is complete occlusion localized as well at the cephalad segment of the common bile duct or at the hepatic duct (Fig. 93).

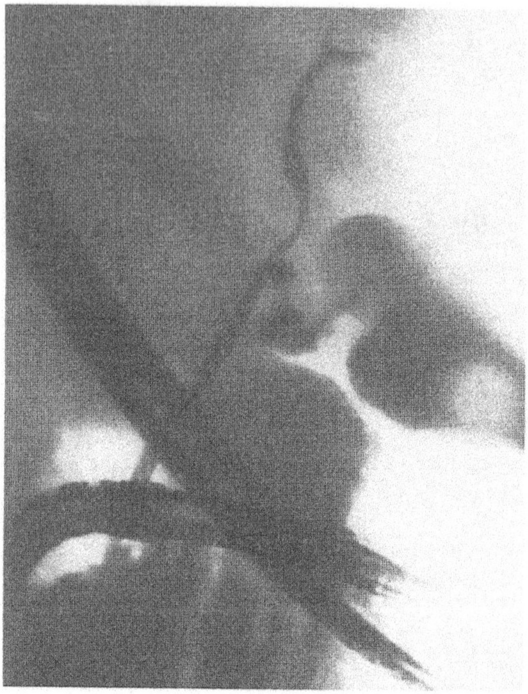

Fig. 93. Intrahepatic biliary carcinoma. Occlusion of branching of hepatic duct. Stenosis of common hepatic duct, of cystic duct, and of infundibulum of gallbladder. Solitary concrement in gallbladder

In such conditions one cannot differentiate carcinoma of the bile ducts from cancer of the porta hepatis. When the proximal segments cannot be visualized, percutaneous transhepatic cholangiography is indicated as a supplementary examination enabling the surgeon to assess the extent of the stricture or stenosis (Geisse et al., 1975; Burwood et al., 1973).

8.5 Stenosis of the Common Bile Duct Secondary to Diseases of Pancreas and Liver

In chronic pancreatitis the common bile duct is affected rather often by the immediate neighborhood of the duct to the pancreatic head. The bile duct is narrowed, showing prestenotic dilatation (Fig. 48). Of 64 patients with chronic pancreatitis, Classen and Demling (1973) found changes in 10 cases. As a rule, the narrowed segment has smooth contours, the stenosis can be sideward or circular. Sometimes, however, the stricture can be eccentric with irregular contours. In such cases differentiation from pancreatic carcinoma by means of ERPC alone is not possible.

In pseudocysts of the pancreas, the common bile duct seems to be affected less often. Of 16 pseudocysts, Romani et al. (1974) only found changes of the bile duct in 2 cases, Stender et al. (1974) report on 3 of 10 pseudocyst cases which presented stenoses or displacement of the common bile duct. The authors observed involvement of the common bile duct in 5 cases out of 28 pseudocysts.

Whether a papillary stenosis, which, according to Classen and Demling (1973), can be found in a high percentage as a coexisting lesion in chronic pancreatitis, should be considered as cause or sequela of chronic pancreatitis, cannot be decided.

Narrowing or even occlusion of the common bile duct secondary to pancreatic cancer, especially if it is localized in the head, can be found even more often than in chronic pancreatitis. Classen and Demling (1973) report on 11 of 16 pancreatic carcinoma cases with stenosis and prestenotic dilatation of the common bile duct (Figs. 70+79). The authors observed these changes 15 times in 47 pancreatic carcinomas. Of 12 carcinomas observed by Stadelmann et al. (1973), the common bile duct was visualized in 6 cases. In all these cases, the bile duct presented a stenosis which in 3 cases was combined with displacement. Romani et al. (1974) found pathologic changes of the common bile duct in 23 pancreatic carcinomas.

The site of the stenosis secondary to carcinoma is identical with that due to chronic pancreatitis. Thus, for differentiation of changes secondary to chronic pancreatitis from changes due to carcinoma, stenosis should never be regarded as an isolated sign but should be judged in connection with the other roentgen features. When the diagnosis of pancreatic carcinoma has been established, involvement of the common bile duct allows one to assess the minimum extent of the tumor indicated by the distance between the changes of the pancreatic duct and the stenosis of the bile duct.

As a rule, involvement of the bile duct signifies inoperability since the tumor has already penetrated beyond the confines of the gland into a neighboring organ.

For the above-mentioned reasons, simultaneous visualization of the pancreatic and the biliary duct system should be tried in all lesions of the pancreas.

Classen and Demling (1973) reported on successful retrograde pancreaticography in relatively rare diseases such as mucoviscidosis and liver cysts. In mucoviscidosis they found cystic dilatations spread all over the duct system. A liver cyst could be partially filled with contrast material through a fistula to the duodenum. Safrany et al. (1974) observed localized, or wide-spread stenoses and variations in caliber of intra- and extrahepatic bile ducts in about half of 20 patients with primary biliary cirrhosis. Further experience will show how these findings and rarified branching are indicative of liver cirrhosis. Complications and syndromes following choledochoduodenostomy, such as fistulae or increased narrowing of the stenosed papillary segment combined with retention of calculi in the retroduodenal blind segment, can generally be detected by upper gastrointestinal barium studies. ERPC should be performed only when this technique fails. Yet, in papillary stenosis, ERPC is always indicated, since the two duct systems can be affected and only this method can clear up the entire symptom complex.

9. Correlation of ERPC with Other Roentgenologic Examinations of the Pancreas

Now that diagnostic efficiency of ERPC in various diseases has largely been demonstrated, its place within the scope of other roentgenologic methods should be examined, as well as the advantages and limits of this technique including its practical use and the various pancreatic diseases.

Annular pancreas is a developmental defect and it presents clinical relevance only when the duodenal lumen is narrowed with consecutive stenotic obstruction. The stenosis may be primary or secondary to inflammatory swelling. Therefore, in this condition the upper gastrointestinal barium study is the most important examination (Table 6). Difficulties in differential diagnosis of duodenal stenoses can justify ERPC for further diagnostic information.

Table 6

Annular pancreas:	Upper gastrointestinal barium study (ERPC)
Acute pancreatitis:	Abdominal plain film, chest survey film
Chronic pancreatitis:	Upper gastrointestinal study combined with hypotonic duodenography, echography, scintigraphy, ERPC, angiography
Pseudocyst:	All examinations, upper gastrointestinal barium study in the beginning
Pancreatic abscess:	Echography, ERPC
Papillary stenosis:	ERPC, transvenous cholangiography, PTC (percutaneous transhepatic cholangiography)
Pancreatic carcinoma:	ERC and angiography (early diagnosis), upper gastrointestinal barium study with hypotonic duodenography, echography and scintigraphy as screening tests
Operability:	Venous phase of angiography, cavography with retroperitoneal venography
Papillary tumor:	Duodenoscopy with forceps and brush biopsy (ERPC)
Insulinoma:	Angiography
Injury to the pancreas:	Echography, angiography, ERPC

This method can demonstrate dystopia and annular course of a duct segment that communicates with the pancreatic head, primarily presenting changes secondary to chronic pancreatitis (Classen et al., 1972).

In *acute hemorrhagic pancreatitis* the patient's poor condition, shock, and peritoneal symptoms do not allow for any invasive method. In this condition the only roentgenologic method that can be indicated for course orientation are abdominal survey plain films and chest films.

In 72% of all cases of *chronic pancreatitis* pathologic changes can be seen in upper gastrointestinal studies (Loeffler et al., 1972), and only in 38% can a reliable diagnosis be established by this technique (Lamarque et al., 1972). Arteriography improves the diagnostic yield 43–71% (Lamarque et al., 1972; Romani et al., 1974 collective statistical studies on 420 cases, Triller et al., 1975; Kramann, 1975; Anacker et al.). On the other hand, in chronic pancreatitis ERPC can lead to a reliable diagnosis in 82–97% (Romani: collective statistic studies on 180 cases; Triller et al., 1975; Kramann, 1975; Anacker et al., 1975). By means of ultrasound studies on 65 cases, from which only 22 could be confirmed, the authors established a true correct diagnosis in 13 cases. A high percentage of cases presenting chronic pancreatitis can be detected by scintigraphy. However, pathologic findings in pancreatic imaging do not allow for a reliable differential diagnosis.

In view of the diagnostic efficiency and also the complication rate, stress to the patient, expenditure of staff, material, and time, it may be useful in cases of suspect chronic pancreatitis to begin with upper gastrointestinal barium studies, including hypotonic duodenography followed by ultrasound echography, and pancreatic scintigraphy. Further diagnostic differentiation can be made by means of ERPC, which may aid the surgeon in planning the operation to be performed and the best suited drainage. If all these examinations cannot rule out uncleared diagnostic problems, arteriography is considered. In chronic pancreatitis indication for arteriography is supplementary and, according to Reuter (1969), only positive findings confirming the diagnostic suspicion should be evaluated. The combination of these roentgenologic examinations yield far more diagnostic information than one can get with only one of these techniques (Classen et al., 1972; Triller et al., 1975; and Anacker et al., 1975). In the authors' case material valuable information that presented essential help in establishing the diagnosis of chronic pancreatitis was yielded by ERPC in 10 cases, by arteriography in 3 cases, and by ultrasonic echography in 2 cases. Romani et al. report on similar results. Of 26 chronic pancreatitis cases that had been examined by ERPC and arteriography, 1 false negative result was observed in ERPC, whereas arteriography failed in 10 cases; thus, the diagnosis could be corrected by ERPC in 9 cases.

Pancreatic pseudocysts containing large quantities of fluid, which have more or less overstepped the confines of the gland, can be detected with sufficient reliability by the orthodox methods. In this condition the upper gastrointestinal barium examination and, if possible, the "extented gastrointestinal examination" with translateral supine and prone views and posteroanterior right and left lateral recumbent views, presents sufficient diagnostic information.

ERPC is the first examination by which *pancreatic abscesses* and *postnecrotic cavities* can be directly visualized provided that the cavity communicates with the duct system so that it can be filled. Indeed, cavities can be detected by ultrasonic echography independent of the existence of a communication of the cavity with the duct system. However, ERPC, while demonstrating the communication of the cavity with the duct system, gives better information as to a more precise localization of the lesion within the gland, thus saving the surgeon time for exploration (Weiss et al., 1972). On the other hand, in view of possible infection of the necrotic cavity, the operation should follow ERPC, within the next 12–24 h. Boijsen (1966), and Tylen and Denker (1973) reported on pancreatic abscesses detected by arteriography. However, arteriograms may give a less graphic picture for surgical intervention. Thus, when pancreatic abscess is suspected, ultrasonic echography might be indicated first. In dubious results, and for better assessments of the draining function of the cavity, ERPC should be performed.

In *pancreatic carcinoma* the diagnostic yield of conventional roentgenographic examinations ranges from 39.5–68% (Berk, 1941; Beeler and Kirklin, 1952; Friman-Dahl, 1961; Wehling et al., 1968; Lamarque et al., 1972). Until 1970 angiography could improve the diagnostic yield up to 64%; in 1975 it reached 76% according to 437 cases from the literature. Among these studies Rösch's results (1973) are outstanding, presenting a total yield of 95%, which are obtained by a superselective technique. According to Romani et al. (1974), the efficiency of ERPC amounts to 95%; in the authors' material of 45 carcinomas, the diagnostic yield of ERPC amounts to 92%. When *the same patients* are submitted to arteriography and ERPC as well, the results demonstrate that ERPC is slightly superior to arteriography. Examinations revealed identical results in the two techniques in 10 of 15 cases. In 4 patients diagnosis was established by ERPC, in 1 patient by arteriography (Anacker et al., 1975). In 13 patients, which had been submitted to this combined examination, Clouse et al. (1975) found an identical diagnostic yield. In 3 other patients, however, cannulation of the papilla failed. In any case, the combination of diagnostic procedures yields more diagnostic information than one method alone (Loeffler et al., 1972; Triller et al., 1975).

Pancreatic scintigraphy can detect pathologic changes in carcinoma as well as in chronic pancreatitis. However, the unspecific changes do not allow further diagnostic differentiation.

The results of ultrasonic echography are promising, but the small number of cases does not yet allow a final judgment.

In carcinoma, apart from the accuracy of the diagnostic method, the possibility of establishing an early diagnosis and to get information as to operability must be taken into consideration. Theoretically, angiography as well as ERPC enables the examiner to detect a carcinoma in an early stage. In a retrospective study, Lunderquist (1965) has detected carcinomas ranging from 0.5–1 cm in size. Since the majority of pancreatic carcinomas arise from the duct system, their early detection is definitely possible and has already been sporadically reported in the literature. As to information concerning operability, angiography is by far superior to ERPC. Involvement of the splenic vessels and of the superior mesenteric vein indicates inoperability. On the other side, inoperability can be suspected in ERPC when the common bile duct is involved.

Apart from these diagnostic qualifications, the usefulness of a technique is determined by its complication rate, technical difficulty, general or individual radiation exposure to the patient, and by the expenditure of staff, material, and time (Table 7).

In contrast to the formerly practiced percutaneous splenoportography, all other current techniques mentioned above present a low and tolerable complication rate. ERPC has high technical difficulties, whereas angiography requires a particularly high amount of staff, material, and time.

Table 7. ERPC compared with angiography in pancreatic carcinoma

Method	Advantages	Disadvantages
ERPC	High diagnostic accuracy early detection (theoretically possible)	High technical difficulties
	Rare information on inoperability	Much discomfort to the patient
	Low complication rate	
Angiography	High diagnostic accuracy; early detection (theoretically possible)	High expenditure of staff, material, and time
	Information on inoperability	High radiation exposure
	Low complication rate Low radiation exposure	

Another shortcoming of angiography is radiation exposure to the patient, which is considerably higher than in ERPC.

With regard to all these factors it seems to be advisable to use ultrasonic echography and scintigraphy first as screening tests followed by ERPC and angiography for precise detection of pancreatic carcinoma (Table 7).

Olsson and Tylen (1971) proved that a *papillary carcinoma* can be demonstrated by angiography. In this condition, ERPC has the advantage that a papillary carcinoma can be diagnosed endoscopically and be confirmed by biopsy. In this condition ERPC is superior to angiography and echography, which does not allow differentiation of papillary carcinoma from carcinoma of the pancreatic head since a papillary carcinoma can be diagnosed endoscopically and be confirmed by biopsy. Hence it follows that in papillary carcinoma, ERPC seems to be the most appropriate technique.

Since in *islet cell carcinoma* the pancreatic duct is almost never involved, ERPC cannot be expected to give positive results. Since the first arteriographic demonstration of an islet cell adenoma by Olsson in 1963, this technique can be regarded as the method of choice, even if only a certain percentage of islet cell tumors are hypervascularized and therewith detectable by arteriography.

An *injury* involving the pancreas can lead to rupture of the parenchyma, arteries, and the duct system. Thus, echography and arteriography as well as ERPC are indicated. By means of echography, posttraumatic escape of pancreatic juice from the duct system and cyst formation can be detected in the same way as in postnectrotic cavities. Rupture of vessels is diagnosed by arteriography, demonstrating lacunary pooling of dye (Geindre et al., 1973) or occlusion of vessels (Hvoijka, 1970). ERPC detects ruptures of the duct system, showing escape of dye from the main duct or the side branches. Echography, while representing least inconvenience to the patient, should precede the other examinations.

10. Conclusion

Unlike the other diagnostic techniques endoscopic retrograde pancreaticocholangiography enables the examiner to visualize directly the glandular structure of the pancreas. As could be expected even before the method was introduced, its diagnostic efficiency presents a certain superiority to other techniques. However, ERPC alone cannot sufficiently cover all diagnostic problems. Further improvement of diagnostic yield can be expected by efficient combination of ERPC with other radiologic and physical techniques, especially with those allowing visualization of the whole gland in combination with better biopsy techniques, and which can give reliable histologic or cytologic confirmation.

References

Abbruzzese, A.A.: Retrograde cholangiography and sclerosing cholangitis. Amer. J. dig. Dis. **19**, 571–574 (1974)

Ammann, R.W., Deyhle, P., Butikofer, E.: Fatal necrotizing pancreatitis after peroral cholangiopancreatography. Gastroenterology **64**, 320 (1973)

Anacker, H.: Die Füllungs- und Entleerungsvorgänge in den Gallenwegen. Fortschr. Röntgenstr. **81**, 142–150 (1954)

Anacker, H.: Röntgenanatomie des Pankreas. Fortschr. Röntgenstr. **94**, 1–13 (1961)

Anacker, H.: Die pathologischen Veränderungen des Pankreasgangsystems im Röntgenbild. Fortschr. Röntgenstr. **96**, 455–470 (1962)

Anacker, H.: Kritische Bewertung der röntgenologischen Untersuchungsmethoden zur Pankreasdiagnostik. Radiologe, **5**, **8**, 312–318 (1965)

Anacker, H.: Anomalien und Variationen des Pankreas. Der Radiologe **7**, 2, 41–52 (1967)

Anacker, H.: Roentgen-anatomy of the pancreas. In: Efficiency and Limits of Radiologic Examination of the Pancreas. Anacker, H., (ed.) Stuttgart: Thieme, 1975; p. 42

Anacker, H., Gaul, A., Kramann, B., Weiss, H.-D., Wiesner, W.: Evaluation of angiography and pancreatography in the radiological diagnosis of pancreatic diseases. In: Demling, L., and Classen, M. (eds.). Endoscopy of the Small Intestine with Retrograde Pancreato-Cholangiography. Stuttgart: Thieme 1973, pp. 64–70

Anacker, H., Weiss, H.-D., Kramann, B.: Die normale und die pathologische Entleerung des Ductus pancreaticus, insbesondere bei der Papillenstenose. Fortschr. Röntgenstr. **118**, 391 (1973)

Anacker, H., Weiss, H.-D., Kramann, B.: Das Pankreaskarzinom im endoskopischen retrograden Pankreatiko-Cholangiogramm. Fortschr. Röntgenstr. **122**, 3, 238–242 (1975)

Anacker, H., Weiss, H.-D., Kramann, B., Rupp, N.: Experience with endoscopic retrograde pancreaticography. Amer. J. Roentgenol. **122**, 375–384 (1974)

Anacker, H., Weiss, H.-D., Kramann, B., Rupp, N., Grünber, G., Lanz, W.: Die Pankreatikographie und ihre Korrelation mit der Angiographie und der Ultrasonographie in der Pankreasdiagnostik. Radiologe **15**, 183–190 (1975)

Anacker, H., Weiss, H.-D., Wiesner, W.: Das pankreatikographische Bild der entzündlichen Pankreasprozesse. Fortschr. Röntgenstr. **117**, 418 (1972)

Anacker, H., Weiss, H.-D., Wiesner, W., Scholze, H.: Die Bedeutung der transduodenalen endoskopischen Pankreatographie. Dtsch. med. Wschr. **95**, 1764–1765 (1971)

Andersson, A., Edström, C., Saltzman, G.-F., Schampi, B.: Concretions in the pancreatic duct diagnosed by Cholangiography. (1968)

Artigas, V.: Sur une Modalité technique de Pancréatographie. J. Radiol. Électrol., 267–268 (1965)

Bartelheimer, H.: Quantitative fraktionierte Pankreas- und Gallensaftuntersuchungen durch Anwendung einer dreläufigen Doppelballonsonde. Dtsch. med. Wschr. **78**, 993 (1953)

Bauerle, H., Grassmann, P.H., Classen, M., Demling, L.: The use of radiographic techniques in gastroenterological endoscopy. Electromedica **4**, 109–114 (1972)

Becker, V.: Bauchspeicheldrüse. In: Spezielle pathologische Anatomie. Doerr, W., Seifert, G., Uehlinger, E. (eds.). Berlin-Heidelberg-New York: Springer-Verlag 1973

Beeler, J. and Kirklin, B.: Roentgenologic findings accompanying carcinoma of pancreas. Am. J. Roentgenol. **67**, 576–584 (1952)
Belsito, A.A., Cramer, G.G., Dickinson, b.P.: Delayed ductal drainage. An endoscopic pancreatographic sign of carcinoma of the head of the pancreas. Amer. J. Roentgenol. **119**, 1, 109–114 (1973)
Bergkvist, A., Seldinger, S.I.: Pancreatic reflux in operative cholangiography in relation to pre- and postoperative pancreatic affection. Acta chir. scand. **114**, 191–196 (1958)
Berk, J.E.: Diagnosis of carcinoma of pancreas. Arch. Int. Med. **68**, 555 (1941)
Bernhard, F.: Die Bedeutung der Cholangiographie für Praxis und Forschung. Chirurg **9**, 201–208 (1937)
Birnstingl, M.: A Study of pancreatography. Brit. J. Surg. **202**, 128–139 (1959)
Boijsen, E., Tylén, U.: Vascular changes in chronic pancreatitis. Acta radiol. (Diagn.) (Stockh.) **12**, 34–48 (1972)
Boijsen, E.: Selective pancreatic angiography. Brit. J. Radiol. **39**, 481 (1966)
Bornschein, W., Weiss, H.-D., Kramann, B.: Das Verhalten der Serum-Lipase-Aktivität bei endoskopischer retrograder Pankreatikographie. Dtsch. med. Wschr. **99**, 20–28 (1974)
Bornschein, W., Weiss, H.-D.: Serum-Lipase-Aktivität und endoskopische retrograde Pankreaticographie bei chronischer Pankreatitis und Pankreasneoplasma. Dtsch. med. Wschr. **100**, 297–308 (1975)
Bücherer, E., Boldt, I., Frommhold, H., Käufer, C.: Die angiographische Diagnostik der Pankreastumoren und der Pankreatitis. Fortschr. Röntgenstr. **115**, 726–741 (1972)
Burwood, R.J., Davies, G.T., Lawrie, B.W., Blumgart, L.H., Salmon, P.R.: Endoscopic retrograde choledocho-pancreatography. Clin. Radiol. **24**, 397–415 (1973)
Campuzano, M., Pitol, A.: Pancreatografia operatoria. Su utilidad clinica. Rev. Invest. clin. **17**, 29–33 (1965)
Christen, T.P.: Zur Technik der Pankreatocholangiographie (PCG). Fortschr. Röntgenstr. **118**, 2, 146–151 (1973)
Chvojka, J.: Ein Beitrag der gezielten Angiographie zur Diagnostik der Pankreasverletzungen. Fortschr. Röntgenstr. **113**, 336–339 (1970)
Classen, M., Anacker, H., Stadelmann, O., Seifert, E., Fritsch, E. von: Diagnose von Tumoren der Papilla Vateri und der Bauchspeicheldrüse durch endoskopisch-radiologische Cholangio-Pankreatikographie. Symposium Radiologicum Pancreatis. München, 1973
Classen, M., Anacker, H., Stadelmann, O., Seifert, E., Fritsch, E. von: The diagnosis of tumours of the papilla of Vater and of the pancreas by endoscopic-radiologic cholangio-pancreaticography (ERCP). In: Efficiency and Limits of Radiologic Examination of the Pancreas. Anacker, H. (ed.). Stuttgart: Thieme 1975 pp. 203–209
Classen, M., Demling, L.: Präoperative Pankreasdiagnostik mit der Duodenoskopie. Chirurg **43**, 247 (1972)
Classen, M., Demling, L.: Retrograde Cholangiographie beim Verschlußikterus. Radiologe **13**, 35–40 (1973)
Classen, M., Hellwig, H., Rösch, W.: Anatomy of the pancreatic duct. A duodenoscopic-radiological study. Endoscopy **5**, 14–17 (1973)
Classen, M., Koch, H., Demling, L.: Diagnostische Bedeutung der endoskopischen Kontrastdarstellung des Pankreasgangsystems. Leber Magen Darm **2**, Nr, 3, 79–81 (1972)
Classen, M., Wenz, W., Fritsch, E.v.: Pankreasdarstellung-Kombination von retrograder Pankreaticographie und Coeliacographie. Dtsch. med. Wschr. **98**, 1524–1526 (1973)
Clouse, M.E., Gregg, J.A., Sedwick, C.E.: Angiography or pancreatography in diagnosis of carcinoma of the pancreas. Radiology **114**, 605–610 (1975)
Cotton, P.B., Beales, J.S.M., Cole, I.A.: Hazards of endoscopic retrograde cholan-

gio-pancreatography. In: Endoscopy of the Small Intestine with Retrograde Pancreato-Cholangiography. Demling, L., Classen, M. (eds.). Stuttgart: Thieme 1973

Cotton, P.B., Beales, J.S.M.: Endoscopic pancreatography in management of relapsing acute pancreatitis. Brit. med. J. **1**, 608–611 (1974)

Cotton, P.B., Salmon, P.R., Blumgart, L.H., Burwood, R.J., Davies, G.T., Lawrie, G.T., Pierce, J.W., Read, A.E.: Cannulation of the papilla of Vater via fiber-duodenoscope. Lancet **1**, 53–58 (1972)

Davenport, H.W.: Physiologie der Verdauung. Stuttgart: Schattauer Verlag 1971, p. 172

Demling, L., Classen, M.: Duodenojejunoskopie. Dtsch. med. Wschr. **95**, 27, 1427–1428 (1970)

Demling, L., Classen, M.: Duodenojejunoscopy, Endoscopy **2**, 115–117 (1970)

Deyhle, P., Fumagalli, J., Paez, C., Jenny, S., Pretet, B., Jenny, M., Ammann, R.: Klinischer Wert der endoskopischen retrograden Pankreato-Cholangiographie. Dtsch. med. Wschr. **97**, 1139–1141 (1972)

Doppman, J., Johnson, R.H.: Reflux pancreatography. Invest. Radiol. **2**, 2, 113–118 (1967)

Doubilet, H., Mulholland, J.H.: Operative contrast visualization of pancreatic disease. In: The Surgical Clinics. Saunders, W.B. (ed.). Philadelphia: Cy., 1956

Doubilet, H., Poppel, M.-H., Mulholland, J.H.: Pancreatography. Technics, principles and observations. Radiology **64**, 325–339 (1955)

Doubilet, H., Poppel, M.H., Mullholland, J.H.: Pancreatography. Ann. N.Y. Acad. Sci. **78**, 829–851 (1959)

Fehr, H.: Fortschr. Röntgenstr. Ein Fall von Pancreas anulare. **101**, 669 (1964)

Felson, B.: Gas Abscess of pancreas. J. Amer. med. Ass. **163**, 637 (1957)

Födisch, H.: Feingewebliche Studien zur Orthologie und Pathologie der Papilla Vateri. Stuttgart: Thieme 1972

Frimann-Dahl, J.: Radiology in tumours of the pancreas. Clin. Radiol. **Vol. XII.** No. 2, 73–79 (April, 1961)

Fritsch, A.: Die Röntgendarstellung des Pankreasganges – eine anatomische Studie. Chirurg **28**, 6, 250 (1957)

Fritsch, A.: Die Bedeutung der Pankreatikographie für die Pankreaschirurgie. Zentralblatt für Chirurgie **28**, 1214 (1962). 79th Conf. d. Dtsch. Ges. f. Chirurgie

Fritsch, E.v., Koch, H., Classen, M.: Retrograde Pankreatikographie. Bewertung von 423 retrograden Pankreatikogrammen. Fortschr. Med. **92**, 241–244 (1974)

Fujita, R., Kumura, F., Hasegawa, Y., Sohma, S., Kidokoro, J.: Endoscopic pancreato-cholangiography. 2nd European Congress of Digestive Endoscopy. Paris, July, 1972

Galvan, A., Klotz, A.P.: Is transduodenal pancreatography ever contraindicated? American Society for Gastrointestinal Endoscopy. Dallas, May, 1972

Gaucher, P., Jeanpierre, R., Watnin, B., Bigard, M., Bas, M., Vicari, F., Laurent, J., Heully, F.: Analyse critique des aspects radiologiques fourni par la Wirsungographie et la cholangiographie per-duodénoscopique chez les malades atteints de pancréatite chronique. 2nd European Congress of Digestive Endoscopy. Paris, July, 1972

Gaylis, H., Gunn, K.: Transduodenale cholangiography. Gynec. Obstet. **100**, 249 (1955)

Geindre, M., Marty, F., Fournet, J., Baudin, Ph., Champetier: Aspects angiographiques des contusions du pancreas. A propos de quatre observations. Ann. Radiol. **16**, 341–347 (1973)

Geisse, G., Melson, G., Tedesco, L., Francis, J., Kelly, J.J., Stanley, R.J.: Stenosing Lesions of the Biliary Tree. Evaluation with endoscopic retrograde cholangiography (ERC) and percutaneous transhepatic cholangiography (PTC). Amer. J. Roentgenol. **123**, 378–385 (1975)

George, P.: Disorders of extrahepatic biliary tree. Clin. Gastroenterol. **2**, 127–146 (1973)

Gomez Oliveros, L., Rhode, M., Rhode, L.: Beobachtungen zu dem funktionellen, muskel-elastischen dynamischen System der Gallenleiter-Bauchspeicheldrüseneinmündung in den Zwölffingerdarm. Morph. Jb. **113**, 13 (1969)

Greenfield, H., Siegel, L.H., Francis, N. de: Attempted visualization of the pancreatic ducts by ampullary reflux. Gastroenterology **29**, 280–284 (1955)

Grimmel, K., Liehr, H., Kasper, H., Kulke, H.: Lipase-Aktivität im Serum nach retrograder transduodenaler Pankreato-Cholangiographie. Dtsch. med. Wschr. **99**, 43–48 (1974)

Gruber, G.B.: Pathologie der Bauchspeicheldrüse. In: Handb. path. Anat. Henke, F., Lubarsch, O. (eds.). Berlin: Springer Vol. V. 1929

Guadagno, N., Mungo, A.: L'importanza della radiologia gastro-intestinale nella diagnosi di cancro del pancreas. Nunt. radiolo. (Firenze) **6**, 472–491 (Giugno 1961)

Gualdi, G., Messe, G.: Aspetti anatomo-radiografici dell'arborizzazione di ordine minore del sistema escretore del pancreas. Nunt. radiol. (Firenze) **3**, 213–230 (1960)

Gualdi, G., Messe, G.: Rilievi anatomo-radiografici sul sistema escretore del pancreas con particolare riferimento ai canali accessori della testa. Nunt. radiol. (Firenze) **25**, 391–412 (1959)

Hara, Y., Ogoshi, K.: Retrograde pancreatography via fiber-duodenoscopy in endoscopy of the small intestine with retrograde pancreato-cholangiography. Demling, L., Classen, M. Stuttgart: Thieme 1973

Harms, E.: Über Druckmessungen im Gallen- und Pankreasgangsystem. Arch. klin. Chir. **147**, 637–654 (1927)

Heitz, F.: Pancréatographie par voie veineuse par excrétion d'érythrosine B chez le chien. Presse méd. **73**, 1815–1818 (1965)

Henry, A., Wollheim, P.: Einige Beobachtungen über das Pancreassekret pflanzenfressender Thiere. Arch. ges. Physiol. **14**, 456–468 (1876–1877)

Hentschel, M.: Variationen der Pankreasgang-Anatomie und Duodenalstumpfverschluß. Der Chirurg **39**, 4, 181–184 (1968)

Herring, P.T., Simpson, S.: The pressure of pancreatic secretion, and the mode of absorption of pancreatic juice after obstruction of the main ducts of the pancreas. Quart. J. Exp. Physiol. **2**, 99–108 (1909)

Herrmann, K.O.: Fortschr. Röntgenstr. **74**, 421 (1951)

Hess, W.: Die chronische Pankreatitis. Vol. 6, pp. 140–150. Bern: Huber 1969

Heully, F., Dornier, R., Gaucher, P., Vicari, F., Bas, M., Laurent, J., Fays, J., Bigard, M.A., Jeanpierre, R.: Expérience de la duodénoscopie. Séminaire de la Societé Internationale d'endoscopie gastrointestinale Karlovy Vary (Tchécoslovaquie), June 6, 1971

Heully, F., Gaucher, P., Laurent, J., Vicari, F., Dornier, R., Bas, M., Fays, J., Jeanpierre, R.: La duodénoscopie. Expérience personnelle. Ann. méd. Nancy **10**, 1533–1540 (1971)

Heully, F., Dornier, R., Gaucher, P., Vicari, F., Bas, M., Laurent, J.: La duodénoscopie. Premiers résultats. – Réunion de la S.M.I.E.R., Hôpital Bichat, Paris, janv. 1971

Hodes, P.J., Pendergrass, E.P., Winston, N.J.: Pancreatic, ductal, and vaterian neoplasms: Their roentgen manifestations. Radiology, **Vol. 62**, 1–15 (1954)

Howard, J.M., Short, F.W.: An evaluation of pancreatography in suspected pancreatic disease. Surg. Gynec. Obstet. **129**, 319–324 (1969)

Hughes, E.S.R. and Kernutt, R.H.: Austr. N. Z. J. Surg. **23**, 223 (1954)

Jacobsson, B., Lanner, L.O., Radberg, C.: The dynamic variability of the choledocho-pancreatico-duodenal junction. Acta radiol. (Stockh.) **52**, 4, 269–281 (1959)

Jeanpierre, R., Léger, L.: Pancréatographie transpapillaire sous duodénoscopie. Chirurgie **97**, 489 (1971)

Jeanpierre, R., Laurent, J., Bas, M., Fays, J., Dornier, R., Bigard, M., Vicari, F., Gaucher, P., Heully, F., avec la collaboration de Merle, M.: Cathétérisme de l'ampoule de Vater au Cours des Examens Duodénoscopiques. Techniques et résultats. Arch. franc. Mal. Appar. dig. Paris **60**, 525–534 (1971)

Kamieth, H.: Die duodenographische Röntgendiagnostik der Papilla Vateri. I. Die normale Papilla Vateri. a. Der Papillenkörper und die Papillenfunktion. Radiologe **10**, 360–363 (1971 a)

Kamieth, H.: Die duodenographische Röntgendiagnostik der Papilla Vateri. I. Die normale Papilla Vateri. b. Die Ampulla Vateri und die Papillenfunktion. Radiologe **10**, 364–367 (1971 b)

Kasugai, T., Kuno, N., Kizu, M., Kobayashi, S., Hattori, K.: Endoscopic pancreatocholangiography. I. The normal endoscopic pancreatocholangiogram. Gastroenterology **63**, 227–234 (1972)

Kasugai, T., Nobuyoshi, K., Kizu, M., Kobayashi, S., Hattori, K.: Endoscopic pancreatocholangiography. II. The pathological endoscopic pancreatocholangiogram. Gastroenterology **63**, 227 (1972)

Kleitsch, W.P.: Anatomy of the pancreas. Arch. Surg. **71**, 795–80 (1955)

Kozu, T.: Duodenoscopic collection of the intraductal pure pancreatic juice and its application to the cytodiagnosis. In: Endoscopy of the Small Intestine with Retrograde Pancreato-Cholangiography. Demling, L., Classen, M. Stuttgart: Thieme 70–73 (1973)

Kozu, T., Classen, M., Koch, H., Demling, L.: Duodenoskopie. Mat. Med. **23**, 287–295 (1971)

Kozu, T.: Fiberduodenoscopic suction of bile and pancreatic juice directly from the papilla of Vater, and the analysis of the acquired fluid in relation to pancreozymin secretin test. Abstracts of 4th Wld Congr. Gastroenterol. 1970

Kozu, T., Oi, I., Suzuki, S., Takamoto, T.: Fiberduodenoscopic observation on the dynamics of the duodenal papilla. Endoscopy **2**, 99 (1970)

Kramann, B., Gullotta, U., Rupp, N., Weiss, H.-D.: Arteriografia pancreaticografia retrograda e sonografia nella diagnosi delle affezioni pancreatiche. IX Congresso dei Radiologi di Cultura Latina Venice, October, 1974

Kramann, B.: A comparative study on duodenoscopic pancreaticography, arteriography and barium meal examination in the diagnosis of chronic pancreatitis. In: Efficiency and Limits of Radiologic Examination of the Pancreas. Anacker, H. (ed.). Stuttgart: Thieme, 209–213, 1975

Kramann, B., Weiss, H.-D.: Differential diagnosis of stenoses of the pancreatic duct system. 3rd Internat. Congr. Gastrointestinal Endoscopy; October 19–21, Mexico-City 1974, p. 164

Kreel, L.: Pancreatic duct calibre and variations on autopsy pancreatography. In: Efficiency and Limits of Radiologic Examination of the Pancreas. Anacker, H. (ed.). Stuttgart: Thieme, 1975, 224–228

Lamarque, J.-L., Ginestie, J.-F., Combes, C., Senac, J.-P.: Aspects Artériographiques des Cancers du Pancréas et des Pancréatites. Confrontations Sémiologiques et Radio-Anatomiques. Ann. radiol. **15**, 697–718 (1972)

Lanz, W.: Unsere Erfahrungen mit der Pankreassonographie. Fortsch. Röntgenstr. **121**, 2, 216–223 (1974)

Lecco, T.M.: Zur Morphologie des Pancreas anulare. S.-B. Akad. Wiss. Wien **119**, 391 (1910)

Ledoux-Lebard, G., Heitz, F., Atlan, H., Rosier, J., Behar, A., Aries, M.: La Pancréatographie par voie veineuse par excrétion d'un produit tétrajodé. Presse méd. **72**, 27, 1579–1582 (1964)

Léger, L.: Images de dilatation du canal de Wirsung. Essai de classification. Presse méd. **69**, 631–633 (1961)

Léger, L., Arway, N.: Pancreatographie pre-opératoire. Presse méd. **35**, 735 (1951)

Legge, D.A., Carlson, H.C., Hoffman, H.N. II: A roentgenologic sign of regional enteritis of the duodenum. Radiology **100**, 37–39 (1971)

Loeffler, P.-G., Schneider, C., Haug, H.P.: Fortschritte in der Diagnostik des Pankreas durch Kombination der röntgenologischen und nuklearmedizinischen Untersuchungsmethoden. Fortschr. Röntgenstr. **117**, 200–206 (1972)

Lunderquist, A.: Angiography in carcinoma of the pancreas. Acta radiol. (Stockh.), Suppl. 235 (1965)

Manegold, B.C.: Endoscopic retrograde pancreaticography (ERPC) in pre- and postoperative pancreatic disease. In: Efficiency and Limits of Radiologic Examination of the Pancreas. Anacker, H. (ed.). Stuttgart: Thieme 1975

Manegold, B.C., Böttger, E., Renner, M.: Maligne Tumoren an den Gallenwegen. Ihre Darstellung im endoskopischen retrograden Cholangiogramm (ERCG). Fortschr. Röntgenstr. **121**, 6, 767–777 (1974)

Mann, C., Foster, J.T.: The secretory pressure of the liver with special reference to absence of the gallbladder. Amer. J. Physiol. **11–12** (1918–1919) p. 278

McCune, S.W., Shorb, E.P., Moscovitz, H.: Endoscopic cannulation of the ampulla of Vater: A preliminary report. Ann. Surg. **167**, 752–756 (1968)

Melvin, E., Clouse, M.E., James, A., Gregg, J.A., Sedgwick, C.E.: Angiography vs. pancreatography in diagnosis of carcinoma of the pancreas. Radiology **114**, 605–610 (1975)

Menguy, R.B., Hallenbeck, G.A., Bollman, J.L., Grindlay, J.H.: Intraductal pressures and sphincteric resistance in canine pancreatic and biliary ducts after various stimuli. Surg. Gynec. Obstet. **106** (1958) 306–320

Mercadier, M., Hepp, J.: Radiologie dans les tumeurs pancréatiques. Ann. Chir. 981–988 (1956a)

Mercadier, M., Hepp, J.: L'apport de l'examen radiologique opératoire au cours du traitement chirurgical des affections pancréatiques. Ann. Chir. **32**, 725–731 (1956)

Miederer, S.E., Löffler, A., Siedek, M., Stadelmann, O.: Die endoskopische retrograde Cholangio-Pankreatographie (E.R.C.P.) als postoperative Untersuchungsmethode. Med. Welt **25**, 1285–1288 (1974)

Millbourn, E.: Calibre and appearance of the pancreatic ducts and relevant clinical problems. Acta chir. scand. **118**, 286–303 (1959/1960)

Mutzenbach, P.: Die superselektive Pankreasangiographie (Technik, Vor- und Nachteile). Röntgenpraxis **24**, 273–284 (1971)

Naatanen, J.F.: Frankf. Zschr. Path. **41**, 198 (1931)

Nabe, R.: Pankreatographie über eine postoperative Pankreashautfistel bei einem medullären Pankreaskopfkarzinom. Fortschr. Röntgenstr. **110**, 5 758–759 (1969)

Nebel, O.T., Fornes, M.F.: Endoscopic Pancreatocholangiography. Amer. J. dig. Dis. **18**, 1042–1050 (1973)

Nette, L.: Radiologisch sichtbare Veränderungen von Pankreasgang und Parenchym bei Pankreaserkrankungen. Dtsch. Röntgenkongreß Baden-Baden 1973

Nette, L., Deyhle, P.: Der Röntgenbefund bei der retrograden Pankreatographie und sein pathologisch-anatomisches Substrat. Radiol. clin. biol. **43**, 328–333 (1974)

Nuboer, J.F.: Studien über das extrahepatische Gallenwegssystem. Der Bau der Muskeln und des elastischen Gewebes in den normalen extrahepatischen Gallenwegen. Frankf. Path. **41**, 198 (1931)

Ogoshi, K., Tobita, Y., Hara, Y.: Endoscopic observation of the duodenum and pancreato-choledochography using duodenofiberscope under direct vision. Gastroenterolog. Endosc. **12**, 83–94 (1970)

Ogoshi, K., Hara, Y.: Retrograde pancreatocholedochography. Japan. J. clin. Radiol. **17**, 455–466 (1972)

Oi, I.: Endoscopic pancreatography by fiberduodenoscope (FDS-Lb). Jap. J. Gastroent. **66**, 880–883 (1969)

Oi, I.: Pancreatography in chronic pancreatitis. In: Endoscopy of the Small Intestine with Retrograde Pancreato-Cholangiography. Demling, L., Classen, M. (eds.). Stuttgart, Thieme 1972, pp. 55–60

Oi, I., Takemoto, T., Nakayama, K.: Fiberduodenoscopy—early diagnosis of cancer of the papilla of Vater. Surgery **67**, 561–565 (1970)

Oi, I.: Duodenoscopy during pancreatic disease. Arch. franc. Mal. Appar. dig. **61**, 349–354 (1972b)

Oi, I., Takemoto, T., Kondo, T.: Fiberduodenoscope: Direct observation of the papilla of Vater. Endoscopy **1**, 3, 101–103 (1969)

Oi, I., Kobayashi, S., Kondo, T.: Endoscopic pancreato-cholangiography. Endoscopy **2**, 103–106 (1970)

Okuda, K., Someya, N., Goto, A., Kunisaki, T., Emura, T., Yasumuto, M., Shimokawa, Y.: Amer. J. Roentgenol. **117**, 437–445 (1973)

Olsson, O., Tylén, U.: Angiography in carcinoma at the papilla of Vater. Acta radiol. (Stockh.) Sweden. 375–386 (1971)

Opie, E.: The anatomy of the pancreas. Am. Med Phila. 996–998 (1903)

Osnes, M., Myren, I.: Endoscopic retrograde cholangio-pancreatography (ERCP) in patients with Billroth II partial gastrectomies. Endoscopy **7**, 227–232 (1975)

Ottenjann, R.: Endoskopische Sondierung der Papilla Vateri.: Dtsch. med. Wschr. **94**, 2347–2348 (1968)

Parry, E.W., Hallenbeck, G.A., Grindlay, J.H.: Pressures in the pancreatic and common ducts. Arch. Surg. **70**, 757 (1955)

Patel, J., Lataste, J.: L'intérêt de la ducto-pancréatographie pour établir la distinction entre pancréatite et cancer. Presse méd. **62**[e] Année, 652–654 (1954)

Pfeffer, R.B., Stasior, O., Hinton, J.W.: The clinical picture of the sequential development of acute haemorrhagie pancreatitis in the dog. Surg. Forum **8**, 765 (1957)

Rabinov, R., Simon, M.: Peroral cannulation of the ampulla of Vater for direct cholangiography and pancreatography. Radiology **85**, 693–697 (1965)

Reuter, S.R., Redman, H.C., Joseph, R.R.: Angiographic findings in pancreatitis. Amer. J. Roentgenol. **107**, 56 (1969)

Reuter, St., R.: Superselective pancreatic angiography. Radiology **92**, 74 (1969)

Rienhoff, W.F. and Lewis, D.: Surgical affections of pancreas met with in John Hopkins Hospital from 1889 to 1932, including report of case of adenoma of islands of Langerhans, and case of pancreatolithiasis. Bull. John Hopkins Hosp. **54**, 386–429 (1934)

Ritter, U.: Untersuchungen zur retrograden Insuffizienz der Papilla Vateri. Gastroenterology **1**, 36–39 (1963)

Robbins, A.H., Messian, R.A., Widrich, W.C., Paul, R.Jr., Norton, R.A., Schimmel, E.N., Ogoshi, K.: Endoscopic pancreatography: An analysis of the radiologic findings in pancreatitis Radiology **113**, 293–296 (November 1974)

Robbins, A.H., Paul, R.E., Jr., Norton, R.A., Schimmel, E.M., Thomas, J.G., Sugarman, H.J.: Detection of malignant disease by peroral retrograde pancreatico-biliary ductography. Amer. J. Roentgenol. **117**, 432–436 (1973)

Rösch, J.: Die „superselektive" viszerale Arteriographie. Fortschr. Röntgenstr. **115**, 718–725 (1972)

Rogers, J.V., Copelanda, A.J., Schroder, J.S., Amerson, A.R.: Sclerosing cholangitis-roentgenographic features. Sh. med. J. (Bgham, Ala.) **65**, 587–594 (1972)

Rohrmann, C.A., Silvis, S.E., Vennes, J.A.: Evaluation of the endoscopic pancreatogram. Radiology **113**, 297–304 (1974)

Romani, S., Oselladore, D., Zacchi, C., Feltrin, G.P., Maggio, C., Ravasini, R., Vio, S., Maffessanti, M., Perelli, R., Drusini, A., Miorro, D.: Considerazioni comparative delle risposte scintigrafiche, arteriografiche e duttografiche ascendenti nella patologia pancreatica. Congresso dei Radiologi di Cultura Latina, Venice 1974

Rosenbaum, H.D., Barker, E.G. Jr., Gibson, D.E., Griffen, B.A., Griffen, W.O. Jr.: Reflux pancreatography. Invest. Radiol. **6**, 321–325 (1971)

Rossi, F.: Accidentale opacizzazione dei dotti pancreatichi in corso di splenoportografia. Presupposti teorici per una dutto-pancreaticografia, percutanea, transplenica in particolari condiziono patologiche. Riv. Radiol. **10**, 497–505 (1970)

Ruppin, H., Amon, R., Ettl, W., Classen, M., Demling, L.: Acute pancreatitis after endoscopic/radiological pancreaticography (ERP). Endoscopy **6**, 94–98 (1974)

Ryan, M.D., Doubilet, H., Mulholland, H.: Observations on biliary-pancreatic dynamics in a normal human. Gastroenterology **13**, 1–8 (1949)

Sáfrány, L.: Endoscopy and retrograde Cholangio-Pancreatography after Billroth II operation. Endoscopy **4**, 4, 198–202 (1972a)

Sáfrány, L.: Duodenoskopie, retrograde Cholangio-Pankreatographie. Schweiz. med. Wschr. **102**, 872–877 (1972b)

Sáfràny, L., Ambrus, C., Barna, L., Büki, B., Magyar, I., Szalay, F.: Veränderungen im retrograden Cholangiogramm bei primär-biliärer Leberzirrhose. Fortschr. Röntgenstr. **120**, 258–263 (1974)

Sanchez san Julian, J., Pascual, A., Megias: La imagen colangiográfica del conducto de Wirsung y su significado. Revista Espanola de las Enfermedades del Aparato Digestivo y de la Nutrición **II**, 3–11 (1952)

Sarasin, R., Leger, L. and Thommen, B.: L'exploration radiologique dans les pancréatites. Rev. int. hépat. **5**, 255–272 (1955)

Sarles, H., Muratore, R., Sarles, J.C. and Guien, Cj.: Ictère, suppuration, stéatorrhée et tolérance glucidique au cours des pancréatites chroniques. Arch. Mal. App. Digestif. **48**, 36–61 (1959)

Schirmer, A.M.: Beitrag zur Geschichte und Anatomie des Pankreas. Inaug.-Diss. (Basel) 1893

Schmieden, V. and Sebening, W.: Arch. Klin. Chir. **148**, 319 (1927)

Seifert, E., Stender, H.St., Sáfrány, L., Lesch, P., Luska, G., Misaki, F.: X-Ray findings of pancreatic cysts diagnosed by endoscopic pancreatocholangiography. Endoscopy **6**, 77–83 (1974)

Silverman, J., Hill, B.J.: Intravenous pancreatography—a negative result. Radiology **81**, 596–597 (1963)

Smanio, T.: Via de acesso ao ducto pancreatic principal. Rev. Med. Cir. S. Paulo **15**, 17–36 (1955)

Sobbe, A., Miederer, S.E., Löffler, A., Stadelmann, O.: Der Stellenwert der gezielten retrograden Cholangiographie in der radiologischen Diagnostik der Gallenwegserkrankungen. Fortschr. Röntgenstr. **122**, 390–398 (1975)

Szeleczky, G., Megyeri, L.: Beiträge zur Morphologie der Gegend des Sphincter Oddi. Langenbeck's Arch. klin. Chir. **305**, 139–149 (1964)

Schmarsow, R.: Röntgenologische Darstellung proximaler biliodigestiver Fisteln. Acta radiol. (Stockh.) **4**, 4, 375–384 (1966)

Stadelmann, O., Deyhle, P., Fumagalli, I., Miederer, S.E., Preter, B., Sobbe, A., Löffler, A.: The efficiency of duodenoscopy in the clinical diagnosis procedure. 2nd European Congress of Digestive Endoscopy. Paris 1972

Stadelmann, O., Sobbe, A., Löffler, A., Miederer, S.E.: Die Bedeutung der retrograden Pankreato-Cholangiographie für die klinische Diagnostik. Fortschr. Röntgenstr. **118**, 4, 377–390 (1973)

Stadelmann, O., Deyhle, P., Löffler, A., Hügel, H., Miederer, S.E., Fumagalli, I.: Endoscopic pancreatography in the diagnosis of tumors. In: Endoscopy of the Small Intestine with Retrograde Pancreato-Cholangiography. Demling, L., Classen, M. (ed.). Stuttgart: Thieme 1972

Stender, H.St., Seifert, E., Misaki, E., Luska, G., Lesch, P.: Veränderungen bei Pankreaszysten im retrograden endoskopischen Choledocho-Pankreatikogramm. Fortschr. Röntgenstr. **120**, 3, 253–258 (1974)

Sterling, J.A.: The common channel for bile and pancreatic ducts. Surg. Gynec. Obstet. **98**, 420 (1954)

Stiller, H.: Ein Beitrag zur röntgenologischen Darstellung des Ductus pancreaticus. Röntgenpraxis, **1**, 18–23 (1948)

Takagi, K.: Study of duodenal fiberscopy III. Stomach and Intestine 103–111 (1970)

Takagi, K., Ikeda, S., Nakagawa, J., Sakaguchi, N., Takahashi, T., Kumakura,

K., Maruyama, M., Someya, N., Nakano, H., Takada, T., Takehoshi, T., Kin, T.: Retrograde pancreatography and cholangiography by fiber duodenoscope. Gastroenterology **59**, 445–452 (1970)

Takagi, K., Ikeda, S., Nakagawa, Y., Kumakura, K., Maruyama, M., Someya, N., Takada, T., Takekoshi, T., Kin, T.: Endoscopic cannulation of the ampulla of Vater. Endoscopy **2**, 107–115 (1970)

Tanaka, H., Ishihara, K., Sakumoto, K., and Kurihara, T.: Results on pancreatographic findings in chronic pancreatitis. In: Endoscopy of the Small Intestine with Retrograde Pancreato-Cholangiography. Demling, L., Classen, M. (eds.). Stuttgart: Thieme 1972

Tatsuzo Kasugai, Nobuyoshi Kuno, Minoru Kizu: Manometric endoscopic retrograde pancreatocholangiography. Technique, significance, and evaluation. Digest. Dis **19**, 485–791 (1974)

Tismer, R., Adler, D., Mies, R., Wehrle, J.: Die angiographische Diagnostik der Insulinome. Leber Magen Darm **3**, 265–272 (1973)

Triller, J., Voegeli, E., Halter, F., Witzel, L., Wanger, F.: Die selektive Pankreasangiographie und retrograde Pankreas-Cholangiographie als Kombinationsuntersuchung. Fortschr. Röntgenstr. **122**, 138–144 (1975)

Tylén, U., Arnesjö, B.: Angiographic diagnosis of inflammatory disease of the pancreas. Acta radiol. (Diagn.) (Stockh.) **14**, 215–240 (1973)

Tylén, U., Dencker, H.: Roentgenologic diagnosis of pancreatic Abscess. Acta radiol. (Stockh.) **14**, 9–16 (1973)

Vondrasek, P., Eberhardt, G.: Endoskopische Druckmessungen mittels Halbleitertechnik. Z. Gastroenterol. **12**, 453–458 (1974)

Vossschulte, K.: Chronische Pankreatitis und primäres Pankreaskarzinom. Langenbeck's Arch. klin. Chir. **301**, 360–371 (1962)

Vossschulte, K.: Chirurgie der chronischen Pankreaserkrankungen. Dtsch. med. Wschr. **86**, 1369 (1961)

Vossschulte, K.: Verfahrenswahl, operative Technik und Nachbehandlung bei chirurgischen Massnahmen am Pankreas. Bruns' Beitr. klin. Chir. **207**, 65 (1963)

Vossschulte, K., Wagner, E.: Chirurgische Massnahmen bei chronischer Pankreatitis. Chirurg **39**, 307–312 (1968)

Waldron II, R.L., Luse, S.A., Wollowick, H.E., Seaman, W.B.: Demonstration of a retrograde pancreatic pathway: Correlation of roentgenographic and electron microscopic studies. Amer. J. Roentgenol. **111**, 695–699 (1971)

Waldron II, R.L., Seaman, W.B., Foster, St.: Reflux pancreatography and distention duodenography in humans. Radiology **104**, 295–300 (1972)

Waldron, R.L. II.: Reflux pancreatography. An evaluation of contrast agents for studying the pancreas. Amer. J. Roentgenol. **104**, 632–640 (1968)

Waldron, II, L., Bragg, G., Daly, J., Seaman, B.: Experimental reflux pancreatography and cholangiography. Radiology **88**, 357–360 (1967)

Waldron II, L., Wollowick, E., Wilson, D.: Experimental reflux pancreatography after intubation of the duodenum per os. Radiology **90**, 338–341 (1968)

Wapshaw, H.: Radiographic and other studies of the biliary and pancreatic ducts. Brit. J. Surg. **43**, 132–141 (1955)

Way, L.W., Sleisinger, M.H.: Postoperative syndromes. In: Gastrointestinal Disease. Sleisinger and Fordtran (eds.). Philadelphia: W.B. Saunders ly., 1973

Wehling, H., Wendenburg, H.H., Matthaes, P.: Das Pankreaskarzinom aus radiologischer und chirurgischer Sicht. Med. Welt. **19**, 1124 (1968)

Weiss, H.-D., Anacker, H., Wiesner, W., Kramann, B.: Duodenoskopische Pankreatikographie – Pankreasangiographie: eine Vergleichsstudie. 4. Kongress für Gastroenterologische Endoskopie. Frankfurt, August 1972. In: „Fortschritte der gastroenterologischen Endoskopie“ **Bd 4**, 1973, S. 133–139

Weiss, H.-D., Anacker, H., Wiesner, W.: Die Technik der Duodenoskopie mit retrograder Pankreato- und Cholangiographie. Fortschr. Röntgenstr. **116**, 517–522 (1972)

Weiss, H.-D., Anacker, H., Wiesner, W., Rupp, N.: Duodenoscopic pancreatography. Radiology **106**, 333–339 (May 1973)

Weiss, H.-D.: Techniques and indications for retrograde Pancreaticography. In: Efficiency and Limits of Radiologic Examination of the Pancreas. Anacker, H. (ed.). Stuttgart: Thieme 1975a, 185–193

Weiss, H.-D.: Endoskopische retrograde Pankreatiko-Cholangiographie (ERPC). In: Aktuelle morphologische Pankreasdiagnostik. Gullotta, U., Rupp, N., Weiss, H.-D., Lanz, W. (eds.): Röntgenpraxis **28**, 6, 125–131 (1975b)

Weiss, H.-D., Anacker, H., Kramann,B.: Die transduodenale, endoskopische retrograde Cholangiographie: Normale und pathologische Befunde der abführenden Gallenwege bei 152 retrograden Cholangiographien. Röntgen-Berichte, **Vol. 3**, 47–61 (1974)

Weiss, H.-D., Anacker, H., Kramann, B., Scholze, H.: The diagnosis of necrotizing pancreatic lesions by means of duodenoscopic pancreatography. Amer. J. Gastroenterol. **64**, 26–33 (1975)

Weiss, H.-D., Kramann, B., Gullotta, U., Rupp, N.: Problèmes du diagnostic differentiel de la sténose du conduit pancréatique surtout en considération du cholédoque. Kongressband IX. Congresso dei Radiologia di Cultura Latina. Venice, October 1974

Weidenhiller, S., Fluegel, H., Rösch, W.: Abrasive cytology of the pancreatic and biliary duct in man. Endoscopy **7**, 72–74 (1975)

Westphal, K.: Die Gallenwegserkrankungen in ihrer Beziehung zur Pankreatitis. München med. Wchnschr. **83**, 1553–1559 (1936)

Whelton, M.J.: Sclerosing cholangitis. Clin. Gastroenterol. **2**, 165–173 (1973)

White, T.T., Elmslie, R.G., Magee, D.F.: Observations on the human intraductal pancreatic pressure. Surg. Gynec. Obstet. **118**, 1043–1045 (1964)

Wulsin, J.H., Siler, V.E.: The intraductal secretory pressure of the pancreas in unanesthetized dogs. Surgery **34**, 9–19 (1953)

Zeus, J.: Discussion in: Endoscopy of the small intestine with retrograde pancreato-cholangiography. Stuttgart: Thieme 42 (1973)

Zsebök, Z., Mészáros, Gy.: Angaben zur chirurgischen und Röntgenanatomie des Pankreas. Acta med. XI, **1**, 139–158 (Budapest 1957)

Zucker, T.F., Newburger, P.G., Berg, B.N.: Further studies on continuous secretion of the pancreas. Proc. Soc. ex. Biol. (N.Y.) **29**, 745 (1932)

Subject Index

Abscess pancreatic 68, 70, 72, 74, 105, 106
acine
  carcinoma arising from acini 87
adenocarcinoma 92
adenoma 79
adenomyosis
  in papillary stenosis 78
age
  influence on caliber of pancreatic main duct 54, 55
anesthesia
  local of the larynx 9, 15
angiography 2, 65, as 105, 106, 107
  chronic pancreatitis 65, 107
  injury to pancreas 109
  insulinoma 105, 109
  pancreatic cancer 91, 105, 106, 107, 108, 109
  papillary carcinoma 108, 109
annular pancreas 56, 57, 105
antifoamer 15

Barium Studies 104
  in anastomosis of biliary tract 96
  chronic pancreatitis 105, 106
  pancreatic cancer 105
  pseudocyst 105
bile duct 1, 4, 5, 6, 11, 13, 14, 20, 22, 25
  anastomoses 96
  anatomy 32, 33, 40, 41, 42, 43
  biliary concrements in chronic pancreatitis
  biliary-duodenal fistula
  cannulation rate 97
  in chronic pancreatitis 60, 62, 63, 64, 69, 72, 102
  emptying 44, 45
  in pancreatic cancer 26, 83, 84, 85, 92, 103
  in papillary stenosis 40, 75, 76, 77, 92, 103
  pressure measurement 46, 47, 49, 51, 53
  stenoses secondary to surgical intervention 99
Billroth I stomach 24
Billroth II stomach 23
  cannulation rate 24
biopsy 24, 109
  device 10, 13
  in papillary cancer 92
bleeding
  contact bleeding in papillary tumor 24
brush biopsy 10, 13, 14, 89, 93, 105

Calculi
  in pancreatic duct system 65, 66, 69
camera 12
cancer biliary 101, 102
cancer pancreatic 1, 2, 24, 25, 42, 93
  diagnostic efficiency of conventional roentgenologic examinations 107
  differential diagnosis 90, 91
  pressure values 51
  symptoms in ERPC pattern 59, 66, 79, 80, 81, 82, 83, 84, 85, 87, 90, 95
cannulation 7, 8, 9, 13, 20, 21, 32, 33, 40, 46, 47
  in Billroth II stomach 24
  in papillary cancer 91, 92, 93
  papillary spasm 22
  peroperative 1
  in postoperative conditions 96
  successful cannulation rate 11, 12
  techniques 20
cardia 15, 16, 17
cavities pancreatic 26, 67, 68, 69, 70, 71, 72
catheter 7, 21
  balloon catheters 3, 4, 5, 6, 13, 45
  with distance markers 12
  metal tipped 13, 48
  pressure measurement 47, 48, 51
cholangiography
  percutaneous transhepatic 97, 98, 105
  peroperative 1, 3, 5, 6, 79
  postoperative 1, 5
  transvenous 6, 7, 25, 76

cholangitis
primary sclerosing 97, 98
secondary sclerosing 97, 98, 99
septic 99
cholecystectomy 25
cholecystokinin 4, 7
choledochoduodenostomy 96, 99, 103
barium Studies 104
cholelithiasis 20, 71
cholostasis 26
complications
fatal complication rate 26, 27
contrast material 1, 4, 14
cyst
dysontogenetic of pancreas 28
cytology 89, 90

Diverticulum duodenal 4, 21, 22
and pancreatic reflux 5, 6
duodenography hypertonic 105, 106
duodenum 3, 4, 7, 14, 15, 17, 18, 19, 20, 31, 44, 51, 52, 56, 57
stenosis in annular pancreas 57

Echography 65, 105, 106, 107, 109
ectasia of pancreatic duct system
in chronic pancreatitis 40, 50, 62, 63, 64
in metastases to pancreas 95
in pancreatic carcinoma 80
in papillary cancer 92
in papillary stenosis 77
emptying phase
in papillary spasm 100
separate phase of pancreatic duct and bile duct 44
emptying time 22
delayed in chronic pancreatitis 26, 59, 60, 62
normal 45
in pancreatic cancer 90
in papillary cancer 92
in papillary stenosis 77, 92
extravasation of contrast medium 69, 70, 71, 72

Fiberduodenoscope
Machida 9, 11
Olympus 9, 10, 11
fluoroscopy 14, 19

Gallbladder 6, 100

Hypophysine
contraction of the gallbladder 6

Injection pressure 4, 5, 22
injury to pancreas 105
islet cell tumor 105
adenoma in ERPC 78
adenoma in peroperative pancreatography 79
carcinoma 109

Jaundice obstructive 26

Kerckring's folds 18, 19, 20, 21

Light source 10, 12
lipase
elevation secondary to ERPC 14, 27, 28, 29
liver
cirrhosis 103
cysts 105

Main duct pancreatic, see Wirsung's duct
malformation pancreatic
annular pancreas 56, 57, 105
cystic malformation of side branches 3, 5
marsupialisation
meperidine 15
mucoviscidosis 105
myxocarcinoma 88, 89
duct changes 87

Necrosis pancreatic 25, 26

Operability 105
in pancreatic carcinoma 90

Pancreaticography 2, 9, 32
after partial pancreatectomy
by direct puncture 1, 7
peroperative 1, 4, 80
transvenous 4, 7
pancreatico-jejunostomy 95
pancreatitis acute 105
acute hemorrhagic 106
secondary to ERPC 30
pancreatitis chronic 1, 2, 25, 57, 63, 65, 80
changes of duct system and duration of history 64
correct diagnosis established by ERPC 65
diagnostic efficiency of barium Studies, echography, scintigraphy 106
different stages 59
differential diagnosis 90

involvement of common bile duct 60, 61, 62
lipase activity following ERPC 27, 28
pressure values 51
pancreatography 2
Papilla of Vater 7, 9, 15, 20, 21, 22, 31, 32, 33, 41, 42, 43, 48, 80
adenoma 79
carcinoma 91, 93, 108, 109
and chronic pancreatitis adenoma 79
spasm 82, 97, 100
stenosis 24, 25, 40, 81, 92, 105, 78
and adenomyosis 92
parenchyma pancreatic
calcifications 65, 66, 67
in chronic pancreatitis 57, 59, 60
opacification 79
opacification in pancreatic cyst 69
overfilling 14, 22, 63
patchy filling in localized inflammation 63
premature opacification 63, 64
puncture 7, 8
peristalsis 17, 19, 20
pressure values
biliary 6, 51, 52
duodenal 4, 52, 53
pancreatic 44, 49, 50, 51
pseudocyst 25, 26, 67, 70, 71, 72, 105
surgical intervention 68
symptoms in ERPC 69
pyloric channel 16, 17, 18, 19

Reflex
vaso-vagal 15
reflux
bilio-pancreatic 1, 3, 4, 5, 6, 75, 78
duodeno-biliary 3
duodeno pancreatic 3, 4
pancreo-biliary 78
relaxers 4

Santorini's duct
anatomical variants 36, 37, 41, 42, 43
in embryonic development 57
scintigraphy 65, 106, 107
secretion 4
side branches of pancreas 9
anatomy 35, 36, 37
in inflammatory disease 59, 61, 63, 66, 69, 70, 72, 90
in pancreatic carcinoma 80, 82, 86, 87, 88, 90
in papillary carcinoma 92
visualization and lipase elevation 29
spasmolytics 20, 22
sphincter of Oddi 3, 31, 32, 33, 44, 45
sphincterotomy 96
splenoportography 108

Triflupromacine 15

Varices oesophageal 26

Wirsung's duct
anatomy 34, 57
inflammatory diseases
occlusion 66, 69, 72, 73
perforation 69, 71, 73
stenosis 66, 60, 69, 76, 77, 78
localized duplication 3, 5
in metastases to pancreas 95
displacement 66, 81, 82, 87, 90
occlusion 80, 81, 82
pancreatic carcinoma
stenosis 59, 66, 79, 80, 81, 83, 84, 85, 87, 90
pressure values 44, 49, 50, 51
stenosis due to aneurism of superior mesenteric artery 66, 68
types of opening 40, 41, 42, 43
width 38, 39, 54, 55

L. DEMLING, M. CLASSEN, P. FRÜHMORGEN

Atlas of Enteroscopy

Endoscopy of the Small and Large Bowel;
Retrograde Cholangio-Pancreatography
With the Collaboration of H. KOCH, H. BAUERLE
Translated from the German and Adapted by K.H. SOERGEL, with the Assistance of H. PEASE
286 figures, most in color. XI, 246 pages. 1975

Contents: Instruments. – Duodenoscopy. – Jejuno-Ileoscopy. – Coloscopy. – Illustrations.

One of the main goals of this atlas is to illustrate recent advances in the new technique of gastroenterological endoscopy. The atlas includes information on the utilization of endoscopy in the upper portion of the small intestine as far as the jejunum, the whole of the colon, parts of the terminal ileum as well as on its initial application in the jejunum and ileum. Only two years ago it was still impossible to make a direct optical examination of these organs. Now inflamed or peptic lesions, such as duodenal ulcers, tumors, diverticula and stenoses can be seen and optically evaluated.
In addition, the atlas describes the completely new visualization of the biliary and pancreatic duct systems from Vater's papilla by means of X-ray contrast media. For the first time the pancreatic duct system has been made accessible to radiological examination. Retrograde endoscopic filling is a decisive step forward in the differential diagnosis of cholelithiasis, this procedure being much less distressing to the patient than percutaneous or laparoscopic cholangiography. In general, the atlas presents endoscopic and radiologic date together with macro- and microscopic pathological anatomy. It describes hitherto uncharted terrain as revealed by endoscopy over the last two years. It is of interest to internal specialists, surgeons, pathologists and all general physicians who derive satisfaction from keeping abreast of the advances of modern medicine.

M.A. MEYERS

Dynamic Radiology of the Abdomen

Normal and Pathologic Anatomy
With a Contribution in Ultrasonography by E. KAZAM
638 figures, including 14 color plates. VI, 351 pages. 1976

Contents: Normal Anatomic Relationships and Variants. – Intraperitoneal Spread of Infections. – Intraperitoneal Spread of Malignancies. – Peritoneography: Normal and Pathologic Anatomy. – The Extraperitoneal Spaces: Normal and Pathologic Anatomy. – The Renointestinal Relationships: Normal and Pathologic Anatomy. – The Duodenocolic Relationships: Normal and Pathologic Anatomy. – Intestinal Effects of Pancreatitits: Spread along Mesentric Planes. – The Small Bowel: Normal and Pathologic Anatomy. – The Colon: Normal and Pathologic Haustral Anatomy. – Pathways of Extrapelvic Spread of Disease.

Full-color anatomic cross-sections of the abdomen and pelvis and detailed computerized transaxial tomography (CTT) scans at corresponding levels are presented in an introductory atlas. The main body of this definitive work focuses on an anatomic and dynamic understanding for the radiologic diagnosis of many common and uncommon abdominal diseases. Emphasis is placed on the pathways and diagnosis of the spread of infection, tumors trauma, and the hemorrhage within the intra- and extraperitoneal spaces.

W. WENZ

Abdominal Angiography

In Collaboration with G. van KAICK, D. BEDUHN, F.-J. ROTH

183 figures, some in color, comprising 351 radiographs and 34 drawings. VIII, 217 pages. 1974

Contents: Introduction and historical review.—Radiologic anatomy of abdominal blood vessels.—Angiographic technique.—The abdominal syndrome and angiography.—Special abdominal angiography.—Frequency of use and diagnostic value of abdominal angiography.—Plates.

This book summarizes the indications for abdominal angiography and describes its practical applications. The technique can be applied routinely, even in small radiography departments. Experience gathered over many years is summed up in tables and figures and the chances of success are critically discussed.

The illustrations include a series of operation sites and preparations, also color-subtraction x-rays, a form first applied to the visceral organs.

N. HASSANI

Ultrasonography of the Abdomen

With a Contribution by R. BARD

215 figures. Approx. 145 pages. 1976

Contents: Principles of Ultrasonography.—Hepatic Sonography.—Splenic Sonography.—Pancreatic Sonography.—Vascular Sonography.—Diaphragmatic Sonography.—Sonography of Ascites.—Sonography in Planning Radiation Therapy.—Retroperitoneal Sonography.—Renal Sonography.

The sophisticated diagnostic information provided by gray scale systems and high resolution real time scanners has made ultrasonic investigation the test of choice in many disorders. The text covers the essential principle of ultrasound physics in a straight forward and comprehensive manner. The practical aspects of scanning techniques are emphasized to permit the reader direct application to daily sonographic procedures. Focus on the upper abdominal organs allows a thorough discussion of sono-pathology of value to the specialist looking for a working knowledge of sonography in his field of interest. Ultrasonically guided biopsy and aspiration methods are described in detail. Currently available ultrasonic scanner's and presently used sonographic techniques are critically reviewed for diagnostic efficacy. Considerable correlation with clinical and pathological features is made.

Springer-Verlag Berlin Heidelberg New York

www.ingramcontent.com/pod-product-compliance
Lightning Source LLC
Chambersburg PA
CBHW080745130926
51338CB00012B/51
9783642810909